CHILDHOOD NEPHROLOGY

Childhood Nephrology

Challenges and Triumphs

MARIA M

Mohammed Altaf Hussain

CONTENTS

TABLE OF CONTENT

Chapter 5: Genetic and Inherited Kidney Disorders
5.1 Understanding Genetic Factors in Pediatric Nephrology
5.2 Challenges in Genetic Counseling
5.3 Triumphs in Genetic Therapies and Interventions

Chapter 6: Pediatric Hypertension
6.1 Identifying and Managing Hypertension in Children
6.2 Challenges in Monitoring Blood Pressure in Pediatric Patients
6.3 Success Stories in Hypertension Management

Chapter 7: Nutrition and Growth in Pediatric Nephrology
7.1 Nutritional Challenges in Pediatric Kidney Patients
7.2 Triumphs in Optimizing Growth and Development

7.3 Multidisciplinary Approaches to Nutrition Management
Chapter 8: Psychosocial Aspects of Pediatric Nephrology
8.1 Impact of Chronic Illness on Pediatric Patients and Families
8.2 Addressing Emotional and Social Challenges
8.3 Success Stories in Coping and Support

Chapter 9: Advances in Pediatric Nephrology Research
9.1 Current Trends in Pediatric Nephrology Research
9.2 Challenges in Translating Research to Clinical Practice
9.3 Future Directions and Potential Triumphs

INTRODUCTION

Youth nephrology, the part of medication committed to the review and treatment of kidney problems in youngsters, remains at the crossing point of difficulties and wins. The creating renal framework in youngsters, mind boggling and powerless, requires fastidious consideration and thoughtfulness regarding guarantee legitimate development and usefulness. Exploring the complicated scene of young life nephrology includes tending to a horde of difficulties, from inherent peculiarities to procured infections, and from demonstrative quandaries to helpful victories. As we dig into the diverse domain of pediatric kidney care, it becomes apparent that the victories accomplished in this field are as fruitful medicines as well as in the nonstop quest for understanding and tending to the extraordinary difficulties that youngsters with kidney problems face.

One of the essential difficulties in youth nephrology emerges from the inborn intricacy of the pediatric renal framework. The creating kidneys go through mind boggling processes that are defenseless to innate irregularities, and deviations from the typical formative direction can prompt a range of renal circumstances. Intrinsic irregularities of the kidney and urinary parcel (CAKUT) address a huge part of pediatric nephrology cases, enveloping a scope of conditions from hydronephrosis to renal agenesis. Understanding the atomic and hereditary premise of these peculiarities is fundamental for unwinding the secrets of renal turn of events and tending to the difficulties introduced by intrinsic kidney problems.

Besides, youth nephrology is set apart by the sensitive equilibrium expected in overseeing gained kidney sicknesses. Kids might confront a different exhibit of conditions, including glomerulonephritis, nephrotic disorder, and hemolytic-uremic disorder, each introducing novel indicative and restorative difficulties. The developing idea of these sicknesses, frequently with unusual courses, requests a nuanced approach that joins clinical keenness with the most recent headways in demonstrative innovations and therapy modalities.

Even with such difficulties, wins arise through fruitful intercessions as well as through a more profound comprehension of the basic systems driving these sicknesses, making ready for additional powerful and customized therapies.

Symptomatic difficulties further highlight the complexities of life as a youngster nephrology. Not at all like grown-ups, kids may not generally express their side effects plainly, making it trying to perceive the basic renal pathology. Early location of kidney problems is critical for starting convenient intercessions and forestalling long haul confusions. Be that as it may, the nuance of side effects in youngsters, combined with the uncommonness of a few pediatric renal circumstances, frequently prompts symptomatic difficulties.

The victories in this domain include the ceaseless refinement of symptomatic apparatuses, including progressed imaging methods, hereditary testing, and biomarker disclosure, to upgrade our capacity to precisely and quickly analyze pediatric kidney problems.

Chasing after wins, the field of experience growing up nephrology isn't restricted to the domains of diagnostics and treatment alone. It envelops a comprehensive methodology that perceives the psychosocial parts of overseeing kidney issues in youngsters. Ongoing kidney infection (CKD) and its treatment can fundamentally influence a kid's personal satisfaction, influencing development, improvement, and everyday exercises. Exploring the psychosocial challenges requires a cooperative exertion including pediatric nephrologists, clinicians, and encouraging groups of people for both the youngster and their loved ones. The victories accomplished in this part of experience growing up nephrology stretch out past clinical results, enveloping the strength and versatility of youthful patients and their families despite ongoing disease.

Wins in youth nephrology likewise manifest in the domain of renal substitution treatment (RRT), which becomes vital in instances of cutting edge kidney illness or disappointment. The coming of pediatric dialysis and kidney transplantation addresses critical achievements, offering a life saver to youngsters confronting the difficulties of end-stage renal infection. Developments in dialysis methods custom fitted for pediatric patients, alongside progressions in immunosuppressive treatments for transplantation, have changed the scene of pediatric nephrology, empowering youngsters to make due as well as flourish in spite of the considerable difficulties presented by kidney disappointment.

Besides, the cooperative endeavors of multidisciplinary groups, including nephrologists, specialists, medical attendants, and social laborers, add to the victories in pediatric kidney transplantation. The fragile equilibrium of immunosuppression, unite observing, and tending to the special difficulties of pediatric beneficiaries requires a planned and extensive methodology. As the field keeps on advancing, the victories in kidney transplantation stretch out to working on long haul results, lessening dismissal rates, and upgrading the general personal satisfaction for pediatric transfer beneficiaries.

The difficulties and wins in youth nephrology are not restricted to the clinical setting alone. Research in pediatric renal medication assumes a urgent part in propelling comprehension we might interpret the fundamental components of kidney illnesses and creating imaginative restorative methodologies. The victories accomplished through research stretch out past individual patient results, forming the eventual fate of pediatric nephrology and affecting worldwide endeavors to address kidney wellbeing in youngsters.

1. **Definition and Scope of Childhood Nephrology**

   Youth nephrology, a particular part of medication, is committed to the review, finding, and treatment of kidney problems explicitly in the pediatric populace. This complex field tends to a different scope of renal circumstances that influence youngsters, going from inborn oddities to procured illnesses, and includes an exhaustive way to deal with dealing with the exceptional difficulties presented by the creating renal framework. The extent of life as a youngster nephrology envelops an expansive exhibit of conditions, demonstrative procedures, helpful mediations, and psychosocial contemplations, making it a pivotal discipline in pediatric medical services.

   At its center, youth nephrology manages the complexities of the pediatric renal framework, a dynamic and creating organ critical for keeping up with liquid and electrolyte balance, circulatory strain guideline, and waste disposal. Not at all like grown-ups, youngsters' kidneys go through quick development and development, and any disturbances in this complex formative cycle can prompt a range of renal problems. The extent of young life nephrology incorporates innate irregularities of the kidney and urinary parcel (CAKUT), which address a critical extent of cases in pediatric nephrology. These oddities, going from underlying irregularities like hydronephrosis to additional serious circumstances, for example, renal agenesis, feature the significance of understanding the sub-atomic and hereditary premise of renal advancement to address difficulties at the actual groundwork of kidney wellbeing in youngsters.

   Notwithstanding intrinsic inconsistencies, youth nephrology stretches out its degree to envelop an extensive variety of procured kidney illnesses that can influence youngsters. Glomerulonephritis, nephrotic disorder, and hemolytic-uremic disorder are among the obtained conditions introducing symptomatic and helpful difficulties in the pediatric populace. The extent of life as a youngster nephrology includes distinguishing and dealing with these circumstances as well as grasping their movement with regards to a creating organ framework. This powerful nature of pediatric kidney sicknesses requires an adaptable and versatile methodology that consolidates clinical skill with headways in demonstrative devices and therapy modalities.

Symptomatic contemplations structure a significant part of life as a youngster nephrology's extension, given the difficulties related with perceiving and deciphering side effects in kids. Dissimilar to grown-ups, youngsters may not generally articulate their side effects plainly, and indications of kidney issues can be unpretentious or vague. The field wrestles with the complexities of early discovery, underlining the significance of recognizing renal circumstances at their incipient stages to forestall long haul difficulties. The extent of experience growing up nephrology subsequently incorporates the persistent refinement of analytic apparatuses, consolidating progressed imaging procedures, hereditary testing, and biomarker disclosure to improve accuracy and practicality in diagnosing pediatric kidney problems.

The interdisciplinary idea of life as a youngster nephrology further enlarges its degree to incorporate psychosocial contemplations basic to the consideration of pediatric patients. Constant kidney infection (CKD) and its treatment can fundamentally influence a kid's personal satisfaction, influencing development, improvement, and in general prosperity. The extent of young life nephrology reaches out past the physiological parts of kidney wellbeing to address the psychosocial challenges looked by youngsters and their families. Pediatric nephrologists work as a team with clinicians, social laborers, and encouraging groups of people to guarantee an all encompassing methodology, perceiving the profound and social elements of overseeing persistent disease in youngsters. This comprehensive extension recognizes the significance of supporting the versatility of pediatric patients and their families all through the direction of kidney infection.

Renal substitution treatment (RRT), a basic part of young life nephrology, becomes essential in instances of cutting edge kidney illness or disappointment. The extent of life as a youngster nephrology in this setting includes the use of pediatric-explicit dialysis strategies and headways in kidney transplantation. Advancements in dialysis mean to make the cycle more okay for youngsters, taking into account their extraordinary physiological and mental necessities. Kidney transplantation in the pediatric populace addresses a victory in the extent of experience growing up nephrology, offering an extraordinary mediation for youngsters confronting end-stage renal sickness. The extension stretches out to the cooperative endeavors of multidisciplinary groups associated with transplantation, accentuating the sensitive equilibrium of immunosuppression, unite observing, and tending to the particular difficulties of pediatric beneficiaries.

Research frames a basic piece of life as a youngster nephrology, growing its degree past clinical practice. Progressing research tries add to a more profound comprehension of the basic components of pediatric kidney sicknesses, driving developments in diagnostics and therapy systems. The extent of experience growing up nephrology research includes hereditary examinations, sub-atomic examinations, and clinical preliminaries pointed toward propelling restorative choices and further developing results for pediatric patients. Through research, adolescence nephrology tends to existing difficulties as well as lays the basis for future victories in the field.

In synopsis, youth nephrology is a particular discipline that characterizes and addresses the one of a kind difficulties related with kidney problems in the pediatric populace. Its degree reaches out from inherent inconsistencies to procured sicknesses, incorporating the complicated formative cycles of the pediatric renal framework. Analytic contemplations, psychosocial parts of care, and progressions in renal substitution treatment add to the thorough extent of life as a youngster nephrology.

Past clinical practice, the field effectively participates in research attempts to extend how we might interpret pediatric kidney illnesses and drive headways that shape the fate of care for youngsters confronting renal difficulties. With its comprehensive methodology and obligation to progressing research, youth nephrology assumes a fundamental part in working on the existences of pediatric patients and guaranteeing their drawn out wellbeing and prosperity.

2. **Importance of Nephrology in Pediatric Care**

The significance of nephrology in pediatric consideration couldn't possibly be more significant, as the kidneys assume a crucial part in keeping up with the fragile equilibrium between liquid and electrolytes, disposing of byproducts, and directing pulse. In the pediatric populace, where the renal framework is as yet creating, the meaning of nephrology turns out to be significantly more articulated. Pediatric nephrologists, represented considerable authority in tending to kidney-related issues in youngsters, are fundamental supporters of the general prosperity of pediatric patients. The unpredictable exchange between the kidneys and different physiological cycles highlights the basic job of nephrology in pediatric consideration.

One of the essential reasons nephrology holds tremendous significance in pediatric consideration is the predominance of inborn irregularities of the kidney and urinary plot (CAKUT) in youngsters. These irregularities, which can go from generally gentle circumstances like hydronephrosis to additional extreme issues like renal agenesis, are a huge focal point of pediatric nephrology. Early ID and mediation in instances of CAKUT are urgent for forestalling long haul difficulties and guaranteeing ideal kidney capability as the kid develops. Nephrologists spend significant time in pediatric consideration assume a vital part in diagnosing and dealing with these innate oddities, underscoring the significance of nephrology in protecting the fundamental parts of kidney wellbeing in youngsters. Additionally, the job of nephrology stretches out to tending to obtained kidney illnesses that can influence youngsters. Conditions like glomerulonephritis, nephrotic disorder, and hemolytic-uremic disorder present remarkable difficulties in the pediatric populace. Pediatric nephrologists carry specific mastery to the finding and the board of these circumstances, taking into account the powerful idea of pediatric kidney infections. The significance of nephrology in this setting lies in giving viable medicines as well as in fitting mediations to oblige the continuous development and advancement of the pediatric renal framework.

The demonstrative abilities of nephrology are of fundamental significance in pediatric consideration. Kids may not generally articulate their side effects plainly, making the acknowledgment of renal issues testing. Nephrologists utilize a scope of demonstrative instruments, including progressed imaging strategies, hereditary testing, and biomarker disclosure, to upgrade the accuracy and idealness of findings. Early location is vital for starting opportune intercessions and forestalling the movement of kidney illnesses.

The significance of nephrology in diagnostics goes past distinguishing explicit circumstances; it includes an extensive comprehension of the developing idea of pediatric kidney issues and the capacity to adjust symptomatic ways to deal with suit the novel necessities of youthful patients.

Nephrology's importance in pediatric consideration is additionally highlighted by its job in tending to the psychosocial parts of kidney sickness in youngsters. Persistent kidney illness (CKD) and its treatment can significantly affect a youngster's personal satisfaction, influencing development, improvement, and everyday exercises. Pediatric nephrologists team up with clinicians, social specialists, and encouraging groups of people to give comprehensive consideration that recognizes the close to home and social components of overseeing persistent sickness in youngsters. The significance of nephrology in this setting lies in cultivating versatility, offering support, and guaranteeing that pediatric patients and their families explore the psychosocial challenges related with kidney sickness with a complete and caring methodology.

Renal substitution treatment (RRT), a basic part of nephrology, becomes fundamental in instances of cutting edge kidney sickness or disappointment. The significance of nephrology in pediatric consideration is apparent in the specific procedures created for pediatric dialysis and kidney transplantation. Developments in dialysis mean to make the cycle more average and compelling for kids, taking into account their remarkable physiological and mental requirements. Pediatric nephrologists assume a significant part in assessing the qualification of youngsters for kidney transplantation, organizing multidisciplinary groups, and guaranteeing the progress of these groundbreaking mediations. The significance of nephrology in the domain of RRT reaches out past quick clinical results; it adds to the drawn out prosperity and personal satisfaction of pediatric patients confronting end-stage renal illness.

Moreover, nephrology's significance in pediatric consideration stretches out to the field of examination. Progressing research attempts add to a more profound comprehension of the sub-atomic and hereditary premise of pediatric kidney sicknesses, driving developments in diagnostics and therapy methodologies. The significance of nephrology in research lies in its capability to shape the fate of pediatric consideration, impacting progressions that further develop results, decrease confusions, and up-grade the general personal satisfaction for youngsters with kidney issues. Nephrology research is necessary to tending to existing difficulties and preparing for wins in the field.

3. **Overview of Challenges Faced in Pediatric Nephrology**

Pediatric nephrology, the particular field devoted to the review and the executives of kidney issues in youngsters, faces a huge number of difficulties that require a nuanced and extensive methodology. From inherent peculiarities to gained infections, and from indicative problems to the intricacies of renal substitution treatment, pediatric nephrologists wrestle with a scope of issues that influence the wellbeing and prosperity of their young patients.

This outline dives into the multi-layered difficulties looked in pediatric nephrology, featuring the complexities of finding, treatment, and the psychosocial aspects of overseeing kidney problems in the pediatric populace.

One of the essential difficulties in pediatric nephrology emerges from inborn peculiarities of the kidney and urinary parcel (CAKUT), which envelop a different range of underlying irregularities influencing the creating renal framework in youngsters. These irregularities can appear as hydronephrosis, renal agenesis, or anomalies in the urinary plot, introducing novel difficulties for analysis and the executives. The complexities of CAKUT request a profound comprehension of the sub-atomic and hereditary variables impacting renal turn of events, as well as a sharp clinical discernment to perceive and address these irregularities right off the bat in a youngster's life. The difficulties in CAKUT stretch out to the likely long haul results, including disabled kidney capability and the gamble of hypertension, underlining the significance of early mediation in pediatric nephrology.

Obtained kidney infections further convolute the scene of pediatric nephrology, with conditions like glomerulonephritis, nephrotic disorder, and hemolytic-uremic condition introducing demonstrative and helpful difficulties. The powerful idea of pediatric kidney illnesses adds intricacy, as these circumstances might have eccentric courses and results. Exploring the difficulties of gained kidney illnesses requires pediatric nephrologists to keep up to date with developing examination, indicative innovations, and treatment modalities to give ideal consideration to their young patients. Also, the uncommonness of a few pediatric renal circumstances presents difficulties concerning mindfulness, opportune determination, and the improvement of proof based treatment draws near.

Symptomatic problems comprise one more critical test in pediatric nephrology, attributable to the inborn challenges in perceiving and deciphering side effects in youngsters. Dissimilar to grown-ups, youngsters may not communicate their side effects plainly, and indications of kidney issues can be unpretentious or vague. Recognizing renal pathology in its beginning phases is basic for starting opportune mediations and forestalling long haul complexities. The difficulties in determination require a wise mix of clinical evaluation, lab examinations, and high level imaging methods. Pediatric nephrologists endeavor to refine demonstrative devices, consolidating hereditary testing and biomarker disclosure, to improve the accuracy and practicality of analyses, tending to the test of early identification in the pediatric populace.

The psychosocial parts of overseeing kidney issues in youngsters present an extraordinary arrangement of difficulties that stretch out past the physiological elements of care. Persistent kidney illness (CKD) and its treatment can essentially influence a kid's personal satisfaction, influencing development, improvement, and everyday exercises. Pediatric nephrologists, as a team with clinicians, social specialists, and encouraging groups of people, should address the profound and social components of overseeing constant sickness in kids.

The difficulties in psychosocial care incorporate supporting the psychological prosperity of pediatric patients, tending to the effect of treatment regimens on their regular routines, and giving assets to families to explore the intricacies of living with a youngster with kidney illness. The all encompassing methodology expected in psychosocial care adds an extra layer of intricacy to the difficulties looked in pediatric nephrology.

Renal substitution treatment (RRT), a basic part of pediatric nephrology, presents its own arrangement of difficulties, especially with regards to the creating pediatric renal framework. Pediatric patients confronting end-stage renal sickness might require dialysis or kidney transplantation for endurance. The difficulties in pediatric dialysis include adjusting procedures to suit the novel physiological and mental requirements of kids. Issues like vascular access, liquid equilibrium, and nourishing help require particular consideration in pediatric dialysis. Kidney transplantation, while offering a groundbreaking mediation, presents difficulties connected with benefactor accessibility, immunosuppression, and long haul join observing in the pediatric populace. The difficulties in RRT highlight the requirement for skill in pediatric nephrology to explore the complexities of these life-supporting mediations.

Moreover, the difficulties looked in pediatric nephrology reach out to the more extensive setting of medical services abberations and admittance to particular consideration. In certain districts, restricted assets and a lack of pediatric nephrologists might add to postpones in determination and treatment. The test of guaranteeing evenhanded admittance to excellent pediatric nephrology care is complex and requires purposeful endeavors at the nearby, public, and worldwide levels. Spanning these holes in access is crucial for address the difficulties looked by youngsters with kidney problems, advancing early mediation, and working on by and large results.

Research in pediatric nephrology is a basic part in tending to existing difficulties and driving development in the field. In any case, research itself isn't without challenges, including restricted financing for pediatric-explicit examinations, the requirement for cooperative endeavors across organizations, and the inborn intricacy of pediatric kidney illnesses. The difficulties in research feature the significance of proceeded with speculation and backing to propel how we might interpret the sub-atomic, hereditary, and clinical parts of pediatric nephrology, eventually adding to the improvement of additional powerful symptomatic and restorative techniques.

4. **Navigating Challenges to Achieve Triumphs**

Exploring the many-sided scene of pediatric nephrology, set apart by a horde of difficulties, requires an immovable obligation to accomplishing wins that go past simple clinical results. From intrinsic inconsistencies to obtained illnesses, and from demonstrative predicaments to the intricacies of renal substitution treatment, the field requests a nuanced and complete methodology.

Even with these difficulties, pediatric nephrologists, medical care experts, and scientists endeavor to address the prompt obstacles as well as to make ready for wins that connote progress, strength, and further developed results for youthful patients.

One of the underlying difficulties experienced in pediatric nephrology lies in the domain of inborn irregularities of the kidney and urinary plot (CAKUT).

The complex formative cycles of the pediatric renal framework lead to a range of underlying irregularities, going from generally gentle circumstances like hydronephrosis to additional serious peculiarities like renal agenesis. Exploring these difficulties includes a profound comprehension of the sub-atomic and hereditary elements impacting renal turn of events. Pediatric nephrologists, frequently in a joint effort with geneticists, pursue disentangling the intricacies of CAKUT to analyze and deal with these irregularities as well as to investigate preventive measures and likely remedial mediations. Wins in this setting emerge from effective medicines as well as from progressions in how we might interpret the fundamental hereditary and sub-atomic premise, opening roads for designated treatments and early mediations.

The difficulties in pediatric nephrology reach out to procured kidney illnesses, where conditions like glomerulonephritis, nephrotic disorder, and hemolytic-uremic disorder might give flighty courses. Exploring these provokes requires pediatric nephrologists to remain at the front of exploration and advancement. Wins arise when the field figures out how to treat these circumstances actually as well as when it propels how we might interpret their pathophysiology, making ready for focused on and customized treatment draws near. The powerful idea of pediatric kidney illnesses requires an adaptable and versatile methodology, and wins in this setting include fitting medicines to the particular necessities of every youthful patient, guaranteeing the most ideal results.

Analytic quandaries present one more arrangement of difficulties in pediatric nephrology, especially given the nuances and vague nature of side effects in youngsters. Early discovery of kidney problems is central for starting opportune intercessions and forestalling long haul confusions. Exploring these symptomatic difficulties includes a prudent mix of clinical intuition and high level indicative instruments. Wins in diagnostics are accomplished when pediatric nephrologists embrace state of the art advances, including hereditary testing and biomarker disclosure, to upgrade the accuracy and speed of findings. Past individual cases, wins in this domain add to a more extensive comprehension of the range of pediatric kidney issues, refining demonstrative rules and calculations for further developed exactness.

The psychosocial parts of overseeing kidney problems in youngsters add a layer of intricacy to pediatric nephrology. Persistent kidney sickness (CKD) and its therapy can essentially influence a kid's personal satisfaction, influencing development, improvement, and everyday exercises. Exploring the difficulties in psychosocial care requires a cooperative and multidisciplinary approach, including pediatric nephrologists, clinicians, social specialists, and encouraging groups of people for both the kid and their loved ones.

Wins in psychosocial care are reflected in better psychological wellness results as well as in the flexibility and versatility of pediatric patients and their families. Past clinical medicines, these victories imply an all encompassing way to deal with pediatric nephrology that recognizes the interconnectedness of physical and profound prosperity.

Renal substitution treatment (RRT), including dialysis and kidney transplantation, presents its own extraordinary difficulties in the pediatric populace. The provokes of adjusting dialysis strategies to suit the physiological and mental necessities of youngsters highlight the significance of specific mastery in pediatric nephrology. Wins in pediatric dialysis are accomplished when the field advances to make the cycle more decent and successful for youthful patients. Kidney transplantation, an extraordinary mediation, presents difficulties connected with giver accessibility, immunosuppression, and long haul unite observing. Wins in transplantation include fruitful medical procedures as well as headways in immunosuppressive treatments, decreased dismissal rates, and worked on long haul results for pediatric transfer beneficiaries. The cooperative endeavors of multidisciplinary groups add to these victories, guaranteeing that pediatric patients get by as well as flourish with relocated kidneys.

Also, the difficulties looked in pediatric nephrology stretch out to the more extensive setting of medical services variations and admittance to particular consideration. Restricted assets, a deficiency of pediatric nephrologists, and differences in medical care framework might add to postpones in conclusion and therapy, especially in specific districts. Exploring these difficulties includes backing, instruction, and cooperative endeavors to guarantee evenhanded admittance to great pediatric nephrology care. Wins in tending to medical care variations are estimated in superior access as well as in upgraded mindfulness, early mediation, and in general better results for pediatric patients confronting kidney-related difficulties.

Research in pediatric nephrology assumes a vital part in exploring difficulties and accomplishing wins in the field. The difficulties of restricted subsidizing for pediatric-explicit examinations, the requirement for cooperative endeavors across organizations, and the intricacy of pediatric kidney illnesses require progressing research tries. Wins in research are reflected in a more profound comprehension of the sub-atomic and hereditary premise of pediatric kidney issues, driving developments in diagnostics and treatment procedures. The exploration scene in pediatric nephrology contributes not exclusively to quick victories in persistent consideration yet additionally to the drawn out progress of the field, molding the fate of pediatric nephrology and further developing results for a long time into the future.

CHAPTER 1

Foundations of Pediatric Nephrology

The groundworks of pediatric nephrology lay on a significant comprehension of the creating renal framework in youngsters, combined with particular information in the determination, the board, and treatment of kidney problems well defined for the pediatric populace. As an unmistakable subspecialty inside the more extensive area of nephrology, pediatric nephrology centers around the extraordinary parts of renal wellbeing in youngsters, enveloping intrinsic peculiarities, obtained sicknesses, symptomatic difficulties, and the psychosocial aspects of care. The underpinnings of pediatric nephrology are based upon a multidisciplinary approach that incorporates clinical mastery, research, and a caring comprehension of the intricate interaction between the creating renal framework and the general prosperity of pediatric patients.

At the center of pediatric nephrology is a top to bottom comprehension of the creating renal framework in kids. The kidneys, essential organs liable for keeping up with liquid and electrolyte balance, pulse guideline, and waste disposal, go through quick development and development during adolescence.

The underpinnings of pediatric nephrology include a thorough handle of the physical, physiological, and sub-atomic parts of the pediatric renal framework. Pediatric nephrologists dive into the complexities of renal turn of events, understanding how deviations from the typical direction can prompt inherent abnormalities of the kidney and urinary plot (CAKUT). This fundamental information is basic for early ID, mediation, and the board of inborn peculiarities, framing the reason for specific pediatric renal consideration.

The groundworks of pediatric nephrology reach out to the range of inborn peculiarities experienced in clinical practice. CAKUT, including many underlying irregularities, comprises a huge focal point of pediatric nephrology. Establishments in this setting include a point by point comprehension of conditions like hydronephrosis, renal agenesis, and obstructive uropathies. Pediatric nephrologists plan to recognize these peculiarities right off the bat in a youngster's life, using imaging review, hereditary testing, and clinical evaluations. The essential information on CAKUT guides restorative mediations as well as structures the reason for progressing investigation into the hereditary and sub-atomic underpinnings of intrinsic kidney problems.

Gained kidney illnesses address one more mainstay of the groundworks of pediatric nephrology. Conditions like glomerulonephritis, nephrotic disorder, and hemolytic-uremic condition might influence youngsters, requiring particular mastery in their conclusion and the board. The establishments include a nuanced comprehension of the pathophysiology, clinical show, and movement of these illnesses with regards to the creating pediatric renal framework. Pediatric nephrologists draw on their central information to tailor treatment methodologies that line up with the interesting necessities of youngsters, taking into account factors like development, improvement, and long haul results.

Analytic establishments in pediatric nephrology are based on the acknowledgment of the difficulties related with distinguishing and deciphering side effects in kids. The establishments include a promise to refining symptomatic devices, using progressed imaging strategies, hereditary testing, and biomarker disclosure. Pediatric nephrologists explore the intricacies of early identification, perceiving that unobtrusive or vague side effects might be demonstrative of hidden renal pathology. The establishments in diagnostics reach out past individual cases, adding to the continuous development of analytic standards and approaches that improve the accuracy and practicality of distinguishing pediatric kidney problems.

The underpinnings of pediatric nephrology likewise incorporate psychosocial contemplations necessary to the consideration of youngsters with kidney issues. Persistent kidney infection (CKD) and its treatment can essentially influence a youngster's personal satisfaction, impacting development, improvement, and everyday exercises. Pediatric nephrologists, as a team with clinicians, social laborers, and encouraging groups of people, lay out starting points for an all encompassing methodology that tends to the close to home and social components of overseeing constant sickness in youngsters.

The establishments in psychosocial care include perceiving the special difficulties looked by pediatric patients and their families and offering extensive help that goes past clinical medicines.

Renal substitution treatment (RRT), including dialysis and kidney transplantation, is an essential part of pediatric nephrology. The establishments in this domain include particular information in adjusting dialysis procedures to suit the physiological and mental requirements of youngsters. Pediatric nephrologists, alongside multidisciplinary groups, lay out starting points for assessing qualification for kidney transplantation, exploring the intricacies of benefactor accessibility, and executing immunosuppressive treatments. The establishments in RRT add to the groundbreaking effect of these mediations on

the existences of youngsters confronting end-stage renal sickness, guaranteeing endurance as well as long haul prosperity.

Research frames a necessary piece of the groundworks of pediatric nephrology, driving headways in figuring out the atomic and hereditary premise of
pediatric kidney sicknesses. The establishments in research include progressing endeavors to unwind the intricacies of innate and gained kidney issues,
adding to advancements in diagnostics and treatment procedures. Pediatric
nephrologists took part in research lay out primary information that shapes
the eventual fate of the field, tending to existing difficulties and preparing for
wins in pediatric nephrology.

The underpinnings of pediatric nephrology stretch out past clinical practice
to include the more extensive setting of medical services incongruities and
admittance to particular consideration. Restricted assets, a lack of pediatric
nephrologists, and territorial differences might add to defers in conclusion and
treatment. The establishments include backing endeavors to address medical
services disparities, advance mindfulness, and guarantee that all kids have
evenhanded admittance to top notch pediatric nephrology care. Establishments in this setting add to further developed admittance, early mediation, and
in general upgraded results for pediatric patients confronting kidney-related
difficulties.

1.1 Historical Perspective

The verifiable point of view of pediatric nephrology reveals a captivating
excursion that reflects the development of clinical information and innovation,
as well as the acknowledgment of the special difficulties related with kidney
problems in youngsters. The foundations of pediatric nephrology follow back to
the mid-twentieth 100 years, and its development as a particular field mirrors
the continuous comprehension of the unmistakable parts of renal wellbeing in
the pediatric populace.

In the ahead of schedule to mid-twentieth 100 years, the investigation of
kidney illnesses basically centered around grown-up populaces, with pediatric
cases frequently treated as downsized forms of grown-up conditions.

Youngsters with kidney problems were overseen by broad pediatricians or
internists, and little consideration was given to the extraordinary parts of renal
wellbeing during youth. This verifiable setting highlights the requirement for a
committed spotlight on pediatric nephrology, as the creating renal framework
in youngsters introduced difficulties and contemplations that varied fundamentally from those in grown-ups.

The proper acknowledgment of pediatric nephrology as a particular subspecialty arose during the 1950s and 1960s. Spearheading doctors and analysts,
perceiving the requirement for particular mastery in tending to kidney problems in youngsters, started to establish the groundwork for the field. The
foundation of pediatric nephrology as a perceived discipline harmonized with

progressions in clinical innovation, like the far reaching accessibility of renal biopsies and the coming of dialysis methods. These mechanical advancements furnished pediatric nephrologists with devices to thoroughly investigate the complexities of pediatric kidney sicknesses more.

One of the milestones in the verifiable improvement of pediatric nephrology was the acknowledgment of intrinsic peculiarities of the kidney and urinary plot (CAKUT) as an unmistakable class of pediatric kidney issues. Preceding this acknowledgment, innate oddities were much of the time thought about inconsistent cases without a bringing together subject. The distinguishing proof of CAKUT as a particular gathering of conditions denoted a defining moment in pediatric nephrology, provoking scientists and clinicians to dive into the hereditary and sub-atomic underpinnings of these irregularities. Understanding the intricacies of CAKUT turned into a foundation in the verifiable development of pediatric nephrology, impacting symptomatic methodologies and helpful mediations.

The 1970s and 1980s saw huge steps in pediatric nephrology, with a rising number of devoted pediatric nephrology units being laid out in clinical bases on the world. This development was resembled by the arrangement of expert associations and social orders explicitly centered around pediatric nephrology, encouraging coordinated effort, schooling, and exploration in the field. The verifiable viewpoint of this time mirrors a shift from a summed up way to deal with kidney problems in youngsters to a more specific and nuanced comprehension of pediatric renal wellbeing.

Progressions in analytic advancements further moved the field of pediatric nephrology forward. Ultrasound imaging, hereditary testing, and modern research center strategies became essential parts of the symptomatic armamentarium, empowering pediatric nephrologists to recognize and describe kidney issues in youngsters with more noteworthy accuracy. The verifiable direction of pediatric nephrology highlights the significance of these analytic headways in unwinding the intricacies of both inborn and obtained kidney illnesses in the pediatric populace.

The authentic story of pediatric nephrology is interlaced with the advancement of renal substitution treatment (RRT) for youngsters confronting endstage renal illness. The improvement of pediatric-explicit dialysis strategies, adjusted to the extraordinary physiological and mental necessities of youngsters, denoted a victory in the verifiable excursion of pediatric nephrology. Moreover, kidney transplantation arose as a groundbreaking mediation during the 1960s, offering a life changing choice for youngsters with cutting edge kidney illness. The authentic point of view of pediatric nephrology mirrors the nonstop refinement of transplantation conventions, enhancements in immunosuppressive treatments, and the cooperative endeavors of multidisciplinary groups devoted to guaranteeing the outcome of kidney transfers in pediatric patients.

The authentic development of pediatric nephrology likewise accentuates the significance of psychosocial contemplations being taken care of by youngsters with kidney problems. As the field developed, pediatric nephrologists perceived the significant effect of persistent kidney illness (CKD) on a youngster's personal satisfaction, development, and improvement. The verifiable viewpoint uncovers a developing accentuation on a comprehensive methodology that includes clinical mediations as well as psychosocial support for pediatric patients and their families. This change in context recognizes the interconnectedness of physical and close to home prosperity in the verifiable story of pediatric nephrology.

Research plays had a significant impact in forming the verifiable direction of pediatric nephrology. Continuous examinations concerning the atomic and hereditary premise of pediatric kidney sicknesses have driven advancements in diagnostics and therapy techniques. The verifiable point of view features the commitments of scientists who have devoted themselves to unwinding the secrets of pediatric nephrology, prompting a more profound comprehension of the fundamental components of both inherent and procured kidney problems. Research has been instrumental in molding the underpinnings of pediatric nephrology, impacting clinical practice and making ready for continuous victories in the field.

The last option part of the twentieth 100 years and the start of the 21st century saw a rising acknowledgment of the worldwide effect of pediatric kidney problems. Worldwide joint efforts, the trading of information and ability, and endeavors to address medical care incongruities have become vital parts of the verifiable account of pediatric nephrology. The verifiable point of view highlights the significance of an aggregate worldwide way to deal with pediatric renal wellbeing, underlining the common obligation to further developing results for youngsters confronting kidney-related difficulties around the world.

1.2 Anatomy and Physiology of Pediatric Kidneys

The life structures and physiology of pediatric kidneys structure the establishment for figuring out the remarkable parts of renal wellbeing in youngsters.

The kidneys, crucial organs liable for keeping up with homeostasis, go through powerful changes during youth, affecting liquid equilibrium, electrolyte guideline, and waste end. This exhaustive investigation of the life systems and physiology of pediatric kidneys digs into the multifaceted designs and works that recognize the creating renal framework in youngsters.

The life systems of pediatric kidneys imparts key similitudes to grown-up kidneys however is described by unmistakable highlights intelligent of the continuous development and development during adolescence. Every kid commonly has two kidneys, arranged in the retroperitoneal space on one or the other side of the spine. The size of pediatric kidneys is proportionate to the youngster's age, with fast development happening in the initial not many long periods of life. The gross physical designs incorporate the renal cortex, medulla, and pelvis, which houses the renal calyces and the renal pelvis.

The renal cortex, the external layer of the kidney, contains nephrons — the practical units answerable for separating blood and creating pee. In pediatric kidneys, the nephron thickness is higher contrasted with grown-up kidneys, mirroring the continuous turn of events and variation to the changing physiological requirements of the developing kid. The renal medulla, arranged further inside the kidney, comprises of renal pyramids and tubules. The medullary designs assume a urgent part in concentrating pee, a cycle essential for keeping up with water balance.

The renal pelvis fills in as a gathering chamber for pee before it channels into the ureters, which transport pee from the kidneys to the bladder. The physical elements of the pediatric renal pelvis are especially pertinent in grasping the inclination of youngsters to specific innate abnormalities of the kidney and urinary lot (CAKUT), like hydronephrosis or ureteropelvic intersection impediment. The creating idea of pediatric kidneys makes them helpless to underlying varieties that might affect urinary waste.

The vascular stockpile to pediatric kidneys is fundamental for their capability and advancement. The renal conduits, fanning out the stomach aorta, supply oxygenated blood to the kidneys, and the renal veins return deoxygenated blood to the substandard vena cava. The complicated organization of veins inside the kidneys works with the filtration of blood through the glomeruli, a cycle that is vital to the kidneys' essential capability of eliminating byproducts and keeping an equilibrium between electrolytes and liquid.

The nephron, the useful unit of the kidney, is a mind boggling structure comprising of the renal corpuscle and renal tubule. The renal corpuscle contains the glomerulus — an organization of vessels — and Bowman's container, which encompasses the glomerulus. In pediatric kidneys, the glomeruli are various and thickly stuffed, mirroring the high nephron thickness normal for the creating renal framework. This thickness adds to the proficient filtration of blood, considering the specific maintenance of fundamental substances and the discharge of byproducts in the pee.

The renal tubule stretches out from Bowman's case and comprises of the proximal tangled tubule, circle of Henle, distal tangled tubule, and associating tubule. The tubules are liable for reabsorbing water and fundamental electrolytes, like sodium and potassium, while discharging abundance solutes and byproducts. The life structures of the renal tubule assumes a pivotal part in the guideline of liquid and electrolyte balance, which is especially essential in the pediatric populace given the unique idea of these boundaries during development and improvement.

Understanding the physiology of pediatric kidneys requires an enthusiasm for the systems associated with glomerular filtration, cylindrical reabsorption, and discharge. Glomerular filtration, the most important phase in pee arrangement, happens as blood goes through the glomeruli. The glomerular filtration rate (GFR), a vital sign of kidney capability, mirrors how much filtrate delivered by the kidneys per unit of time. In pediatric kidneys, GFR is impacted by elements, for example, age, body surface region, and development of renal capability, making it a unique boundary that advances over the course of growing up.

Rounded reabsorption and emission happen in the renal tubules and are basic for keeping up with the harmony between electrolytes and liquid. In pediatric kidneys, the effectiveness of these cycles is finely tuned to help the quick development and improvement normal for youth. Reabsorption dominatingly happens in the proximal tangled tubule, where water and solutes are reabsorbed once again into the circulatory system. The circle of Henle assumes a vital part in concentrating pee, with the length and capability of this portion impacting the kidney's capacity to monitor water.

The distal tangled tubule and interfacing tubule further manage electrolyte balance through particular reabsorption and discharge. Sodium reabsorption is a critical cycle in keeping up with extracellular liquid volume and pulse. The physiology of pediatric kidneys includes many-sided hormonal guideline, including the activity of antidiuretic chemical (ADH), aldosterone, and the renin-angiotensin-aldosterone framework. These hormonal components assume a vital part in answering changes in hydration status, electrolyte equilibrium, and circulatory strain, guaranteeing the steadiness of inside conditions in the creating youngster.

The responsiveness of pediatric kidneys to hormonal signs is exemplified by their capacity to adjust to changing dietary salt admission. In babies and small kids, the youthfulness of renal tubules might bring about diminished sodium reabsorption, making them more helpless to sodium misfortune in the pee. This physiological part of pediatric kidneys features the requirement for a reasonable methodology in overseeing liquid and electrolyte irregular characteristics, particularly with regards to diseases or ailments that might affect renal capability.

The physical and physiological parts of pediatric kidneys add to the comprehension of specific one of a kind clinical contemplations in pediatric nephrology.

For instance, the expanded nephron thickness in pediatric kidneys might present a level of flexibility, considering utilitarian pay despite intense putdowns or injury. Nonetheless, it likewise underlines the weakness of pediatric kidneys to formative anomalies and the potential for long haul outcomes in the event that legitimate working is compromised.

Intrinsic abnormalities of the kidney and urinary parcel (CAKUT), going from primary varieties to complex deformities, are intently attached to the life systems and improvement of pediatric kidneys. Understanding the typical formative cycles helps with perceiving and dealing with these oddities, underlining the significance of early location and mediation to forestall difficulties and save kidney capability. Problems, for example, vesicoureteral reflux, hydronephrosis, and renal dysplasia are among the different range of CAKUT that pediatric nephrologists experience in clinical practice.

1.3 Common Pediatric Renal Disorders

Pediatric nephrology envelops a different cluster of renal problems that can influence youngsters from outset through immaturity. Understanding these problems is pivotal for pediatric nephrologists, medical services experts, and guardians the same, as early location and mediation are in many cases key to relieving long haul confusions. This exhaustive investigation dives into normal pediatric renal problems, crossing intrinsic irregularities, gained conditions, and issues that manifest over the course of growing up.

Inherent inconsistencies of the kidney and urinary lot (CAKUT) address a general class of underlying irregularities that emerge during fetal turn of events. Hydronephrosis, described by the expansion of the renal pelvis and calyces, is a typical CAKUT. It frequently results from a block in the urinary lot, for example, vesicoureteral reflux (VUR) or ureteropelvic intersection deterrent (UPJO). Hydronephrosis can be recognized prenatally through antenatal ultrasound, taking into account early assessment and intercession. In instances of VUR, where pee streams in reverse from the bladder to the kidneys, youngsters might be at an expanded gamble of urinary plot diseases (UTIs). Opportune recognizable proof and the board of VUR are significant to forestall intermittent UTIs and potential kidney harm.

Renal agenesis, an interesting innate irregularity, includes the shortfall of one or both kidneys. One-sided renal agenesis frequently stays asymptomatic, with the contralateral kidney making up for its nonattendance. Notwithstanding, reciprocal renal agenesis is contrary with life, regularly bringing about stillbirth or neonatal passing. Multicystic dysplastic kidney (MCDK) is one more intrinsic problem portrayed by non-working cystic kidneys, frequently distinguished prenatally. Much of the time, MCDK doesn't need mediation, as the unaffected kidney can satisfactorily uphold renal capability.

Polycystic kidney illness (PKD), containing autosomal passive polycystic kidney sickness (ARPKD) and autosomal predominant polycystic kidney illness (ADPKD), addresses a gathering of hereditary issues described by the development of liquid filled sores in the kidneys. ARPKD ordinarily gives in outset augmented kidneys, hypertension, and liver contribution. Conversely, ADPKD, which will in general show later in youth or pre-adulthood, can prompt moderate renal debilitation. Hereditary testing assumes a significant part in affirming the determination and directing the administration of PKD.

Nephrotic condition is a gathering of problems portrayed by expanded porousness of the glomerular filtration boundary, prompting huge protein-uria, hypoalbuminemia, edema, and hyperlipidemia. Negligible change sickness (MCD) is the most widely recognized reason for nephrotic disorder in kids. Regardless of the name, the glomeruli in MCD seem typical under light microscopy. Corticosteroids are the backbone of treatment for MCD, and most of kids answer well to this treatment. Different types of nephrotic disorder, for example, central segmental glomerulosclerosis (FSGS) and membranous nephropathy, may require more forceful administration and convey a gamble of movement to ongoing kidney sickness (CKD).

Intense poststreptococcal glomerulonephritis (APSGN) is a resistant inter-ceded problem that commonly follows a streptococcal contamination, like strep throat or impetigo. It frequently gives hematuria, proteinuria, hypertension, and edema. While most instances of APSGN resolve precipitously, a few kids might foster extreme confusions, underlining the significance of brief acknowl-edgment and strong consideration. The frequency of APSGN has diminished in evolved nations however stays a worry in locales with restricted admittance to medical care and unfortunate disinfection.

Hemolytic-uremic disorder (HUS) is a group of three of microangiopathic hemolytic weakness, thrombocytopenia, and intense kidney injury. The most widely recognized structure, frequently connected with Shiga poison deliver-ing Escherichia coli (STEC) diseases, fundamentally influences small kids. HUS can prompt serious complexities, including neurological inclusion and kidney disappointment. The board includes strong consideration, including liquid and electrolyte the executives, and a few cases might profit from plasmapheresis.

Urinary plot contaminations (UTIs) are normal in youngsters and can prompt pyelonephritis, a bacterial disease of the kidneys. Small kids, particularly those with innate abnormalities, are at an expanded gamble of UTIs. Brief analysis and fitting anti-microbial treatment are fundamental to forestall the spread of disease and potential kidney harm. Vesicoureteral reflux (VUR), referenced prior with regards to CAKUT, is a typical hidden factor in repetitive UTIs. Void-ing cystourethrography (VCUG) is frequently used to assess VUR and guide the board choices.

Henoch-Schönlein purpura (HSP) is a fundamental vasculitis that can influ-ence the kidneys, skin, joints, and gastrointestinal parcel. While the etiology of HSP isn't completely perceived, it frequently follows an upper respiratory lot disease.

Renal inclusion can appear as glomerulonephritis, prompting hematuria and proteinuria. Most instances of HSP resolve immediately, however a few youngsters might foster industrious renal infection, stressing the requirement for close observing and strong consideration.

Ongoing kidney sickness (CKD) in youngsters can result from different basic circumstances, including inherent abnormalities, glomerular illnesses, and acquired messes. The movement of CKD can prompt end-stage renal infection (ESRD), requiring renal substitution treatment like dialysis or kidney transplantation. The effect of CKD on development, advancement, and generally personal satisfaction highlights the significance of early identification and complete administration systems.

Renal calculi, or kidney stones, however more uncommon in youngsters contrasted with grown-ups, can happen and introduce novel difficulties. Lack of hydration, metabolic problems, and physical irregularities might add to stone arrangement. The clinical show can incorporate hematuria, flank torment, and urinary side effects. The board includes torment control, hydration, and addressing the fundamental variables adding to stone arrangement. Dietary alterations and drugs might be prescribed to forestall repeat.

Acquired renal cylindrical problems, like Bartter disorder and Gitelman condition, disturb electrolyte balance and can prompt unusual liquid and salt dealing with in the kidneys. Bartter condition regularly gives in earliest stages or youth polyuria, polydipsia, and electrolyte anomalies. Gitelman condition, milder than Bartter disorder, regularly shows later in youth or immaturity. The executives includes tending to electrolyte irregular characteristics and giving steady consideration.

The administration of normal pediatric renal problems requires a multidisciplinary approach, including pediatric nephrologists, pediatricians, urologists, and other medical care experts. Early conclusion through a mix of clinical assessment, research center tests, imaging review, and, now and again, hereditary testing, is basic for starting convenient intercessions and forestalling long haul intricacies. Treatment procedures fluctuate contingent upon the particular issue however may incorporate drugs, dietary adjustments, and, now and again, careful intercessions.

1. **Congenital Anomalies**

    Innate peculiarities of the kidney and urinary parcel (CAKUT) comprise a different gathering of underlying irregularities that emerge during fetal turn of events, influencing the kidneys and related urinary designs. These oddities range from gentle circumstances that might negligibly affect kidney capability to additional serious mutations that can prompt critical wellbeing challenges. Understanding the range of innate oddities is critical for pediatric nephrologists, medical care experts, and guardians, as early identification and mediation assume a significant part in improving results.

Hydronephrosis, portrayed by the widening of the renal pelvis and calyces, is perhaps of the most well-known innate abnormality. It frequently results from a hindrance in the urinary plot, blocking the typical progression of pee. The check can happen at different places, including the ureteropelvic intersection (UPJ), ureterovesical intersection (UVJ), or inside the actual ureter. Antenatal ultrasound has upset the early discovery of hydronephrosis during pregnancy, taking into account opportune assessment and intercession postnatally.

Vesicoureteral reflux (VUR) is another normal innate peculiarity where pee streams in reverse from the bladder into the ureters and, now and again, up to the kidneys. This condition expands the gamble of urinary plot diseases (UTIs) and presents possible dangers to kidney wellbeing. The seriousness of VUR is evaluated, with higher grades demonstrating more huge reflux. Voiding cystourethrography (VCUG) is frequently utilized to evaluate the presence and level of VUR, directing administration choices to forestall repetitive UTIs and safeguard renal capability.

Renal agenesis, an uncommon innate peculiarity, includes the shortfall of one or both kidneys. One-sided renal agenesis, where one kidney is missing, frequently slips through the cracks as the contralateral kidney can repay enough. Conversely, reciprocal renal agenesis, the shortfall of both kidneys, is contrary with life and commonly brings about stillbirth or neonatal passing. Hereditary elements and ecological impacts during early fetal advancement add to the event of renal agenesis.

Multicystic dysplastic kidney (MCDK) is portrayed by the presence of non-working cystic kidneys. This innate peculiarity frequently appears as a coincidental tracking down on pre-birth ultrasound. While MCDK doesn't need dynamic mediation by and large, as the unaffected kidney can keep up with ordinary renal capability, close checking is fundamental to guarantee legitimate development and improvement. The condition may precipitously determine over the long haul.

Polycystic kidney sickness (PKD) contains a gathering of hereditary issues portrayed by the development of liquid filled pimples in the kidneys. Autosomal passive polycystic kidney sickness (ARPKD) normally gives in outset amplified kidneys, hypertension, and liver contribution. Autosomal prevailing polycystic kidney sickness (ADPKD) will in general show later in youth or puberty, prompting moderate renal debilitation. Hereditary testing assumes a significant part in affirming the finding and directing the administration of PKD, which might include strong consideration, prescriptions, and, in extreme cases, renal substitution treatment.

As a feature of the range of CAKUT, back urethral valves (PUV) are a block inside the urethra that transcendently influences male babies. This innate peculiarity obstructs typical pee stream, prompting expansion of the bladder and urinary lot. PUV can bring about critical complexities, including hindered kidney capability and bladder brokenness. Early determination and careful intercession are essential to alleviate long haul results and safeguard renal wellbeing.

Anorectal mutations, a gathering of innate oddities influencing the rear-end and rectum, can likewise be related with urological irregularities, including vesicoureteral reflux or hydronephrosis. The complicated interaction of urological and anorectal designs highlights the significance of a thorough assessment when intrinsic peculiarities are thought. Multidisciplinary joint effort including pediatric nephrologists, urologists, and pediatric specialists is fundamental for ideal administration.

The comprehension and the executives of CAKUT reach out past the neonatal period, as certain peculiarities might become obvious later in youth. Horseshoe kidney, a condition where the lower shafts of both kidneys are intertwined, is one such inconsistency. While it may not be guaranteed to influence kidney capability, people with a horseshoe kidney might be at a marginally higher gamble of specific inconveniences, for example, kidney stones or contaminations. Ordinary observing and resolving likely issues as they emerge add to the general prosperity of people with this inherent abnormality.

As pediatric nephrology propels, the investigation of the hereditary and sub-atomic premise of CAKUT turns out to be progressively critical. Propels in hereditary testing advances empower a more profound comprehension of the hidden systems, preparing for customized medication and designated mediations. The mind boggling connection among hereditary qualities and inborn irregularities underlines the advancing idea of pediatric nephrology and the potential for creative ways to deal with determination and treatment.

2. **Acquired Kidney Diseases**

Obtained kidney sicknesses in youngsters envelop a different exhibit of conditions that might result from contaminations, immune system issues, or other foundational diseases. Not at all like innate oddities, obtained kidney infections foster after birth and can appear at any phase of young life. Understanding these circumstances is fundamental for pediatric nephrologists, medical care experts, and guardians, as ideal determination and mediation assume a basic part in dealing with these problems and saving kidney capability.

Nephrotic condition is a typical procured kidney jumble portrayed by expanded porousness of the glomerular filtration hindrance, prompting critical proteinuria, hypoalbuminemia, edema, and hyperlipidemia. Negligible change illness (MCD) is the most continuous reason for nephrotic disorder in kids.

Notwithstanding the name, the glomeruli in MCD seem ordinary under light microscopy. Corticosteroids, explicitly prednisone, are the essential treatment for MCD, and most of youngsters answer well to this treatment. Notwithstanding, a few cases might be steroid-safe or as often as possible backslide, requiring extra intercessions.

Central segmental glomerulosclerosis (FSGS) is one more type of nephrotic disorder portrayed by scarring (sclerosis) in unambiguous locales (fragments) of the kidney's separating units (glomeruli).

FSGS can result from hereditary transformations, contaminations, or auxiliary to other ailments. The clinical course of FSGS shifts, and the board might include immunosuppressive treatments, including corticosteroids, immunosuppressants, and angiotensin-changing over catalyst (Expert) inhibitors or angiotensin II receptor blockers (ARBs) to oversee circulatory strain and diminish proteinuria.

Membranous nephropathy is described by the thickening of the glomerular storm cellar layer, prompting proteinuria. It is a safe interceded problem, and keeping in mind that it can happen at whatever stage in life, it is less normal in kids than in grown-ups. The basic reason for membranous nephropathy might be idiopathic or auxiliary to contaminations, immune system illnesses, or openness to specific drugs. Treatment methodologies might include immunosuppressive drugs and strong consideration.

Intense poststreptococcal glomerulonephritis (APSGN) is a safe intervened problem that regularly follows a streptococcal disease, like strep throat or impetigo. It frequently gives hematuria, proteinuria, hypertension, and edema. While most instances of APSGN resolve precipitously, a few youngsters might foster serious entanglements, stressing the significance of brief acknowledgment and strong consideration. The occurrence of APSGN has diminished in evolved nations yet stays a worry in districts with restricted admittance to medical care and unfortunate sterilization.

Hemolytic-uremic disorder (HUS) is a set of three of microangiopathic hemolytic sickliness, thrombocytopenia, and intense kidney injury. The most well-known structure, frequently connected with Shiga poison creating Escherichia coli (STEC) contaminations, principally influences small kids. HUS can prompt extreme inconveniences, including neurological contribution and kidney disappointment. The board includes strong consideration, including liquid and electrolyte the executives, and a few cases might profit from plasmapheresis.

Intense kidney injury (AKI) in youngsters might result from different causes, including diseases, parchedness, prescriptions, or fundamental sicknesses. Early acknowledgment and the board are essential to forestall inconveniences and safeguard kidney capability. The basic reason for AKI guides therapy systems, which might incorporate tending to liquid and electrolyte awkward nature, ending nephrotoxic drugs, and dealing with the essential ailment.

Urinary plot diseases (UTIs) are normal in youngsters and can prompt pyelo-nephritis, a bacterial contamination of the kidneys. Small kids, particularly those with intrinsic irregularities, are at an expanded gamble of UTIs. Brief finding and suitable anti-microbial treatment are fundamental to forestall the spread of disease and potential kidney harm. Vesicoureteral reflux (VUR), referenced prior with regards to inherent irregularities, is a typical fundamental variable in repetitive UTIs. Voiding cystourethrography (VCUG) is frequently used to assess VUR and guide the board choices.

Henoch-Schönlein purpura (HSP) is a foundational vasculitis that can influence the kidneys, skin, joints, and gastrointestinal parcel. While the etiology of HSP isn't completely perceived, it frequently follows an upper respiratory parcel contamination. Renal contribution can appear as glomerulonephritis, prompting hematuria and proteinuria. Most instances of HSP resolve precipitously, however a few youngsters might foster industrious renal illness, underscoring the requirement for close checking and steady consideration.

Ongoing kidney sickness (CKD) in youngsters can result from different hidden conditions, including inherent oddities, glomerular illnesses, and acquired messes. The movement of CKD can prompt end-stage renal infection (ESRD), requiring renal substitution treatment like dialysis or kidney transplantation. The effect of CKD on development, improvement, and in general personal satisfaction highlights the significance of early discovery and complete administration methodologies.

Renal calculi, or kidney stones, however more uncommon in youngsters contrasted with grown-ups, can happen and introduce novel difficulties. Drying out, metabolic problems, and physical irregularities might add to stone arrangement. The clinical show can incorporate hematuria, flank torment, and urinary side effects. The board includes torment control, hydration, and addressing the hidden elements adding to stone development. Dietary changes and prescriptions might be prescribed to forestall repeat.

CHAPTER 2

Diagnosis and Evaluation

Diagnosing and assessing kidney problems in youngsters is a diverse cycle that includes a mix of clinical evaluation, lab examinations, imaging review, and, at times, hereditary testing. The complicated idea of pediatric nephrology requires a complete way to deal with precisely recognize the hidden reasons for kidney issues and guide suitable mediations. This investigation will dive into the symptomatic and evaluative parts of pediatric kidney problems, underscoring the significance of a multidisciplinary approach in conveying ideal consideration.

Clinical assessment is much of the time the beginning stage in the determination of pediatric kidney problems. Side effects like hematuria, proteinuria, edema, hypertension, or urinary lot diseases might provoke a medical services proficient, commonly a pediatrician or family doctor, to start further examinations. An exhaustive clinical history, including a family background of kidney issues, birth history, and a definite record of side effects, helps guide the indicative interaction. Actual assessment might uncover indications of liquid maintenance, raised pulse, or development irregularities, giving significant clinical bits of knowledge.

Research center examinations assume a urgent part in surveying kidney capability and distinguishing irregularities characteristic of explicit kidney issues. Urinalysis is a principal demonstrative device that assesses the presence of blood, protein, or different irregularities in the pee. Hematuria, for instance, may propose glomerular or urinary parcel contribution, while proteinuria is a vital marker in conditions, for example, nephrotic disorder. Infinitesimal assessment of urinary residue can additionally refine the symptomatic interaction by uncovering the kind of cells or projects present, giving signs to the fundamental pathology.

Blood tests are necessary to surveying generally kidney capability and distinguishing markers of explicit kidney problems. Serum creatinine and blood urea nitrogen (BUN) levels mirror the kidneys' capacity to channel byproducts from the blood. Raised levels might show debilitated kidney capability. Serum electrolyte levels, including sodium, potassium, and calcium, are firmly checked to evaluate and oversee electrolyte uneven characters that frequently go with kidney problems. Furthermore, blood tests might incorporate markers like enemy of atomic antibodies (ANA) or against twofold abandoned DNA (dsDNA) antibodies to evaluate for immune system conditions that can influence the kidneys.

High level imaging studies are regularly utilized to envision the kidneys and urinary parcel, giving basic data about their construction and capability. Renal ultrasound is a harmless imaging methodology that can evaluate kidney size, shape, and the presence of irregularities or impediments. It is especially valuable in the assessment of inherent oddities, hydronephrosis, or cystic kidney illnesses. Voiding cystourethrography (VCUG) is a particular imaging procedure that evaluates vesicoureteral reflux (VUR), a typical worry in youngsters with urinary plot contaminations.

Figured tomography (CT) examines and attractive reverberation imaging (X-ray) are more definite imaging modalities that might be used in unambiguous cases, for example, evaluating complex renal life systems, recognizing masses or cancers, or portraying cystic sores. These imaging studies give three-layered perspectives on the kidneys and encompassing designs, helping with the finding and careful anticipating specific circumstances.

Renal biopsy is a symptomatic technique that includes the extraction of a little tissue test from the kidneys for tiny assessment. This obtrusive method is normally saved for situations where the hidden reason for kidney illness isn't clear from painless assessments. Renal biopsy can give important bits of knowledge into the particular histopathological changes happening in the kidneys, directing treatment choices and guess. Be that as it may, it isn't without chances, and the choice to continue with a renal biopsy is painstakingly weighed against expected benefits, particularly in pediatric patients.

Hereditary testing has become progressively significant in the finding of pediatric kidney issues, particularly those with a genetic part. Progresses in genomic medication consider the ID of explicit hereditary changes related with conditions, for example, polycystic kidney sickness (PKD), Alport disorder, or certain innate abnormalities. Hereditary testing might be vital for affirming a finding, directing treatment choices, and surveying the gamble of illness movement in families with a background marked by genetic kidney issues.

Practical appraisals, for example, the estimation of glomerular filtration rate (GFR) or explicit pee protein markers, add to the assessment of kidney capability and sickness movement. GFR is a critical mark of by and large kidney capability, and its estimation gives experiences into the seriousness of kidney disability. The assessment of GFR is especially important in surveying persistent kidney illness (CKD) and directing administration procedures. Protein markers, for example, urinary egg whites to-creatinine proportion (ACR), are utilized to measure proteinuria, helping with the determination and checking of conditions like nephrotic disorder.

The assessment of circulatory strain is an essential part of evaluating kidney wellbeing, as hypertension is both a reason and result of kidney problems. Constant or extreme hypertension might bring up doubt of basic kidney sickness, and circulatory strain observing is a vital part of overseeing conditions like glomerulonephritis or renovascular infection. Overseeing pulse actually is fundamental in easing back the movement of kidney illness and forestalling confusions like cardiovascular occasions.

In the domain of pediatric nephrology, the exceptional contemplations of developing kids require a customized and patient-focused way to deal with finding and assessment. The effect of kidney issues on development, improvement, and by and large personal satisfaction highlights the significance of early identification and opportune intercession. Pediatric nephrologists, working as a team with pediatricians, radiologists, hereditary guides, and different subject matter experts, assume a focal part in guaranteeing an exhaustive and individualized demonstrative cycle.

The multidisciplinary idea of pediatric nephrology is exemplified in the administration of complicated cases, where contribution from experts in hereditary qualities, urology, immunology, and radiology might be fundamental. Continuous examination and mechanical progressions persistently improve the demonstrative abilities in pediatric nephrology, giving open doors to prior and more exact distinguishing proof of kidney problems.

2.1 Screening and Diagnostic Techniques

Screening and symptomatic procedures assume a urgent part in the early recognizable proof and complete evaluation of pediatric kidney issues.

The powerful idea of pediatric nephrology requires a smart and individualized way to deal with screening, considering variables, for example, age, risk factors, and introducing side effects. This investigation will dive into different screening and analytic procedures utilized in pediatric nephrology, accentuating their importance in advancing early discovery and compelling administration.

1. **Clinical Assessment and History:**
   Clinical assessment and getting a definite clinical history act as essential strides in the evaluating system for pediatric kidney problems. Side effects like hematuria, proteinuria, edema, hypertension, or repetitive urinary plot diseases (UTIs) may raise doubt and brief further examination. An intensive comprehension of the kid's clinical history, including pre-birth and birth history, family background of kidney problems, and

any significant openness to drugs or poisons, gives important setting to resulting symptomatic evaluations.

2. **Urinalysis:**
Urinalysis is a foundation in the underlying evaluation of kidney capability. This basic and harmless test examines the physical, substance, and tiny properties of pee. The presence of hematuria, proteinuria, or anomalies in urinary dregs can give basic experiences into the fundamental pathology. Minute assessment of pee might uncover red platelets, white platelets, or projects, directing the indicative cycle. Urinalysis is many times a piece of routine well-youngster visits and can act as an early evaluating device for kidney problems.

3. **Blood Tests:**
Blood tests are fundamental for evaluating generally kidney capability and recognizing explicit markers characteristic of kidney problems. Serum creatinine and blood urea nitrogen (BUN) levels mirror the kidneys' capacity to channel side-effects from the blood. Raised levels might propose disabled kidney capability. Serum electrolyte levels, including sodium, potassium, and calcium, are firmly observed to survey and oversee electrolyte uneven characters regularly connected with kidney problems. Extra blood tests might incorporate markers for immune system conditions, like enemy of atomic antibodies (ANA) or hostile to twofold abandoned DNA (dsDNA) antibodies, which are important in immune system interceded kidney sicknesses.

4. **Pulse Estimation:**
Pulse estimation is a critical part of both screening and continuous checking in pediatric nephrology. Hypertension can be both a reason and result of kidney problems, and its initial discovery is fundamental in forestalling complexities. Pulse percentiles in view old enough, sex, and level are utilized to evaluate and arrange hypertension in youngsters. Customary pulse observing is especially significant in conditions like glomerulonephritis, renovascular sickness, or hypertension-related kidney harm.

5. **Renal Ultrasound:**
Renal ultrasound is a harmless imaging methodology that gives important data about the size, shape, and primary trustworthiness of the kidneys and urinary parcel. It is many times utilized as a first-line imaging concentrate on in the assessment of intrinsic peculiarities, hydronephrosis, or cystic kidney illnesses. Renal ultrasound is especially valuable in kids because of its absence of ionizing radiation and capacity to be performed without sedation.

6. **Voiding Cystourethrography (VCUG):**
Voiding cystourethrography is a specific imaging strategy used to evaluate vesicoureteral reflux (VUR), a condition where pee streams in reverse

from the bladder into the ureters and, at times, up to the kidneys. VCUG includes the presentation of a differentiation color into the bladder, and imaging is performed during voiding. This methodology recognizes the presence and grade of VUR, directing administration choices, particularly in kids with repetitive UTIs.

7. **Processed Tomography (CT) and Attractive Reverberation Imaging (X-ray):**

In specific cases, more itemized imaging concentrates, for example, CT outputs or X-rays might be utilized to picture the kidneys and encompassing designs with higher accuracy. CT examines utilize X-beams to make cross-sectional pictures, while X-rays utilize strong magnets and radio waves. These imaging modalities are especially important in surveying complex renal life systems, distinguishing masses or growths, and describing cystic sores. Nonetheless, their utilization is painstakingly thought of, considering variables, for example, the youngster's age, the potential for ionizing radiation with CT examines, and the requirement for sedation.

8. **Hereditary Testing:**

Headways in genomic medication have worked with the utilization of hereditary testing in pediatric nephrology, particularly in cases with a thought genetic part. Hereditary testing can distinguish explicit changes related with conditions, for example, polycystic kidney illness (PKD), Alport disorder, or certain intrinsic peculiarities. It is instrumental in affirming a finding, directing treatment choices, and surveying the gamble of sickness movement in families with a background marked by genetic kidney problems.

9. **Renal Biopsy:**

Renal biopsy is an intrusive technique that includes the extraction of a little tissue test from the kidneys for minuscule assessment. While not a normal screening device, it is utilized when the hidden reason for kidney infection isn't obvious from painless assessments. Renal biopsy gives important histopathological bits of knowledge, assisting with recognizing explicit kidney infections, guide treatment choices, and foresee visualization. The choice to play out a renal biopsy is painstakingly weighed against expected gambles, particularly in pediatric patients.

10. **Utilitarian Appraisals:**

Useful appraisals add to the assessment of kidney capability and sickness movement. The estimation of glomerular filtration rate (GFR), a critical sign of by and large kidney capability, gives bits of knowledge into the seriousness of kidney disability. Assessing GFR is especially significant in evaluating ongoing kidney illness (CKD) and directing administration techniques. Protein markers, for example, urinary egg whites to-creatinine proportion (ACR), evaluate proteinuria, helping with the finding and observing of conditions like nephrotic disorder.

11. **Demonstrative Imaging for Urinary Stones:**
In situations where urinary stones are thought, demonstrative imaging, for example, non-contrast CT filters or renal ultrasound might be utilized to picture the presence, size, and area of stones. These examinations assist with directing treatment choices, including the selection of intercessions, for example, lithotripsy or careful stone expulsion.

12. **Mobile Circulatory strain Checking:**

For kids with thought or analyzed hypertension, mobile circulatory strain observing (ABPM) might be utilized for a more thorough evaluation. ABPM includes wearing a convenient pulse screen north of a 24-hour time frame, giving a more precise portrayal of circulatory strain varieties in a youngster's regular routine. This strategy is especially valuable in separating between white coat hypertension and supported hypertension.

The coordination of these screening and analytic procedures in pediatric nephrology mirrors the intricacy and variety of kidney issues in youngsters. The decision of explicit tests is directed by the clinical show, side effects, and thought fundamental causes. Furthermore, the age and formative phase of the kid are considered to fit the symptomatic way to deal with their novel requirements.

Multidisciplinary cooperation is fundamental in the screening and determination of pediatric kidney problems. Pediatric nephrologists, pediatricians, radiologists, hereditary guides, and different experts cooperate to decipher discoveries, lay out a conclusive determination, and figure out a thorough treatment plan. Early recognition through viable screening methodologies is urgent for starting ideal mediations, upgrading results, and safeguarding kidney capability in youngsters confronting renal difficulties.

2.2 Importance of Early Detection

The significance of early recognition in pediatric nephrology couldn't possibly be more significant, as opportune distinguishing proof of kidney issues fundamentally impacts treatment results, long haul visualization, and in general personal satisfaction for impacted youngsters.

Early location is a basic part of complete medical care, and with regards to pediatric nephrology, it assumes a crucial part in tending to innate irregularities, obtained kidney illnesses, and different renal problems that might appear during youth.

1. **Early Discovery of Innate Inconsistencies:**
Intrinsic inconsistencies of the kidney and urinary parcel (CAKUT) address

a huge classification of conditions that can influence kidney wellbeing from birth. Early location of these oddities is many times worked with by pre-birth ultrasound, permitting medical care suppliers to distinguish underlying anomalies in the creating fetal kidneys. Ideal acknowledgment of conditions like hydronephrosis, vesicoureteral reflux (VUR), or multicystic dysplastic kidney (MCDK) empowers medical services experts to quickly start post pregnancy assessments and mediations.

For instance, recognizing high-grade VUR right off the bat in a youngster's life considers mediations to forestall repetitive urinary plot contaminations (UTIs) and potential kidney harm. Early recognition of CAKUT establishes the groundwork for proper administration procedures, which might incorporate checking, prescriptions, and, at times, careful mediations. The objective is to upgrade kidney capability, forestall intricacies, and guarantee the youngster's general prosperity from the earliest phases of life.

2. **Convenient Acknowledgment of Procured Kidney Illnesses:**
   Gained kidney illnesses in youngsters, for example, nephrotic disorder, glomerulonephritis, or urinary parcel diseases (UTIs), can have assorted etiologies and clinical introductions. Early location of these circumstances is pivotal for starting designated treatments and forestalling the movement of kidney harm.

   On account of nephrotic condition, early distinguishing proof through clinical assessment and research center tests considers brief inception of treatment, frequently including corticosteroids. This convenient intercession can prompt a positive reaction and decrease the gamble of entanglements related with delayed proteinuria and edema.

   Likewise, the opportune acknowledgment of intense poststreptococcal glomerulonephritis (APSGN) it is fundamental to follow a streptococcal contamination. Early steady consideration can alleviate the gamble of difficulties, like hypertensive emergencies or serious kidney injury. Early finding and fitting anti-microbial treatment for UTIs in youngsters assist with forestalling the spread of contamination and limit the gamble of rising diseases that could prompt pyelonephritis and ensuing kidney harm.

3. **The board of Hereditary and Acquired Kidney Issues:**
   Hereditary and acquired kidney issues, for example, polycystic kidney infection (PKD) or Alport condition, frequently have an inherited part.

   Early recognition through hereditary testing permits medical care suppliers to distinguish people in danger inside families with a background marked by these issues. Hereditary advising can give important data about the legacy design, expected signs, and the probability of illness movement.

   On account of PKD, for example, early recognition through hereditary testing takes into consideration observing and the executives techniques that can assist with easing back the movement of the illness. Distinguishing people with Alport disorder right off the bat in life empowers opportune mediations to oversee side effects and moderate the gamble of difficulties like hearing misfortune and kidney disappointment.

4. **Avoidance of Confusions and Movement:**
Early recognition assumes a focal part in forestalling complexities related with kidney issues and limiting the movement of renal disability. For instance, in youngsters with constant kidney illness (CKD), early distinguishing proof considers the execution of procedures to oversee circulatory strain, improve sustenance, and address explicit complexities related with renal brokenness.

Convenient mediation with regards to CKD might incorporate dietary changes, prescription administration, and, at times, renal substitution treatment. Early location of CKD additionally empowers medical care suppliers to address the effect of renal brokenness on development and advancement, guaranteeing that kids get suitable help and intercessions to upgrade their general wellbeing.

5. **Improving Personal satisfaction:**
The meaning of early recognition stretches out past clinical administration; it significantly influences the general personal satisfaction for youngsters confronting kidney problems. By distinguishing conditions early, medical services suppliers can tailor mediations to limit interruptions to ordinary youth exercises, school participation, and social connections.

Youngsters with kidney problems frequently face remarkable difficulties, including dietary limitations, medicine the executives, and likely hospitalizations. Early location takes into consideration the execution of procedures to help the kid's personal prosperity, including psychosocial backing, instruction, and contribution of particular medical care experts who figure out the special requirements of pediatric patients.

6. **Working with Multidisciplinary Care:**
The multidisciplinary idea of pediatric nephrology stresses the significance of early discovery in working with cooperation among medical care experts. Early ID takes into consideration the commitment of a different group of subject matter experts, including pediatric nephrologists, pediatricians, urologists, hereditary guides, dietitians, and social laborers. This cooperative methodology guarantees that the kid gets complete consideration that tends to not just the clinical parts of the kidney issue yet additionally the psychosocial and formative requirements.

7. **Monetary Effect:**
Early discovery can have positive monetary ramifications by possibly lessening the general medical care costs related with overseeing progressed

kidney sickness and its inconveniences. Forestalling the movement of kidney issues to end-stage renal sickness (ESRD) through early intercessions, for example, pulse the executives and dietary changes, can prompt better wellbeing results and possibly decline the requirement for expensive mediations like renal substitution treatment.

8. **Examination and Advances in Treatment:**
Early discovery adds to progressing research endeavors and the improvement of creative treatment approaches in pediatric nephrology. By distinguishing patients from the get-go over their illness, analysts can concentrate on the regular history of different kidney problems, investigate possible biomarkers, and test novel helpful mediations. This constant pattern of examination and clinical practice encourages headways in figuring out, finding, and treatment, eventually helping people in the future of youngsters with kidney problems.

9. **General Wellbeing Effect:**

Advancing early discovery lines up with more extensive general wellbeing drives pointed toward forestalling and overseeing constant circumstances in the pediatric populace. By bringing issues to light about the signs and side effects of kidney problems, empowering routine screenings, and encouraging a proactive way to deal with medical services, general wellbeing efforts can add to the early ID of renal difficulties in youngsters.

2.3 Challenges in Accurate Diagnosis

Precise conclusion is a foundation of successful medical services, and in the domain of pediatric nephrology, it presents extraordinary difficulties that medical services experts should explore. From intrinsic peculiarities to obtained kidney sicknesses, the perplexing idea of the pediatric renal framework presents intricacies in finding that require a complete and nuanced approach. This investigation will dive into the difficulties experienced in precisely diagnosing kidney issues in youngsters, revealing insight into the multi-layered factors that add to the intricacy of pediatric nephrology.

1. **Vague Side effects and Variable Introductions:**
One of the principal challenges in pediatric nephrology lies in the vague idea of side effects related with kidney problems. Youngsters might give unclear side effects like weakness, unfortunate craving, or crabbiness, which can be credited to a bunch of fundamental causes. In addition, the introduction of kidney issues can differ broadly, even among youngsters with a similar fundamental condition.
For instance, glomerulonephritis, a gathering of resistant intervened kidney sicknesses, may appear with side effects going from hematuria and

proteinuria to edema and hypertension. The fluctuation in symptomatology requires a fastidious clinical assessment and a wise determination of demonstrative tests to unwind the particular idea of the renal test.

2. **Restricted Correspondence in Small kids:**
   Correspondence obstructions represent a huge test in pediatric nephrology, especially in more youthful kids who might come up short on capacity to precisely explain their side effects. Newborn children and babies might communicate uneasiness or trouble through crying or changes in conduct, making it provoking for medical services suppliers to pinpoint the wellspring of the issue. This impediment in viable correspondence elevates the dependence on clinical perceptions, parental information, and symptomatic devices to unravel the hidden kidney-related issues.

3. **Covering Introductions with Other Pediatric Circumstances:**
   Kidney issues frequently share covering introductions with other pediatric circumstances, further confusing the analytic interaction. For example, the side effects of nephrotic disorder, like proteinuria and edema, can be at first confused with other normal youth illnesses. Recognizing renal and non-renal reasons for side effects requires an exhaustive examination, frequently including lab tests, imaging review, and in some cases obtrusive systems like renal biopsy.

4. **Demonstrative Difficulties in Children and Babies:**
   The neonatal and baby populaces present special analytic difficulties because of their weakness and restricted capacity to convey side effects. Intrinsic abnormalities of the kidney and urinary plot (CAKUT), which might be asymptomatic upon entering the world, can show later in earliest stages or youth. The dependence on pre-birth ultrasound for early discovery adds one more layer of intricacy, as not all inconsistencies are clear during fetal turn of events. Thusly, the neonatal period requires cautious checking and a high record of doubt for conditions that might turn out to be clinically clear as the kid develops.

5. **Absence of Mindfulness and Instruction:**
   Restricted mindfulness and comprehension of pediatric kidney problems among medical care suppliers, guardians, and the overall population add to postponed or missed analyze. Kidney sicknesses in youngsters may not generally be top of psyche, prompting a likely defer in looking for clinical consideration. Bringing issues to light about the signs and side effects of kidney problems, particularly with regards to routine pediatric consideration, is critical for encouraging early acknowledgment and opportune mediation.

6. **Heterogeneity of Pediatric Kidney Problems:**
   The heterogeneity of pediatric kidney issues presents an imposing test in finding. The range of conditions includes intrinsic irregularities,

glomerular illnesses, tubulointerstitial messes, and innate kidney sicknesses, each with its remarkable clinical elements and analytic contemplations. Exploring this heterogeneity requires a far reaching comprehension of the different exhibit of pediatric kidney problems and the capacity to tailor symptomatic methodologies in view of the particular qualities of each condition.

7. **Demonstrative Imaging Limits in Kids:**
While demonstrative imaging, for example, renal ultrasound, CT outputs, and X-rays, assumes a significant part in assessing kidney design and capability, there are intrinsic limits in the pediatric populace. Radiation openness, particularly in rehashed CT checks, raises worries about expected long haul gambles, especially in kids with constant circumstances requiring progressing observing. Adjusting the demonstrative utility of imaging with the need to limit radiation openness is a continuous test in pediatric nephrology.

8. **Obtrusive Indicative Systems:**
In specific cases, getting a conclusive determination might require obtrusive systems like renal biopsy. Playing out a renal biopsy in a youngster implies cautious thought of the dangers and advantages, as well as the potential for uneasiness and tension for both the kid and their parental figures. Finding some kind of harmony between getting fundamental demonstrative data and limiting the obtrusiveness of techniques is a fragile part of pediatric nephrology practice.

9. **Challenges in Deciphering Lab Results:**
Deciphering research facility brings about the setting of pediatric kidney problems requires a nuanced comprehension old enough unambiguous reference reaches and varieties in lab boundaries. Typical qualities for creatinine, blood urea nitrogen (BUN), and other renal capability markers fluctuate as youngsters develop and create. Inability to represent age-related contrasts might prompt distortion of results and, accordingly, challenges in showing up at an exact determination.

10. **Hereditary and Atomic Intricacy:**
The rising accentuation on understanding the hereditary and atomic premise of pediatric kidney problems adds one more layer of intricacy to the demonstrative scene. Hereditary testing, while significant in affirming specific judgments, acquaints difficulties related with the distinguishing proof of pathogenic variations, the understanding of hereditary information, and the coordination of hereditary discoveries into clinical administration.

11. **Financial Elements and Medical services Incongruities:**
Financial elements and medical care differences can affect the demonstrative excursion of youngsters with kidney problems. Restricted admittance

to medical services assets, postponed admittance to specialty care, and differences in wellbeing proficiency might add to defers in finding and the commencement of fitting mediations. Tending to these abberations is fundamental for guaranteeing evenhanded admittance to convenient and precise indicative assessments for all youngsters, paying little heed to financial foundation.

12. **Long haul Checking and Follow-Up Difficulties:**

When a finding is laid out, the difficulties reach out into long haul observing and follow-up. Pediatric nephrology frequently includes the administration of constant circumstances, and continuous observing is vital for track infection movement, change treatment techniques, and address arising intricacies. Planning long haul care, particularly for conditions like ongoing kidney infection (CKD), requires a cooperative methodology including the youngster, their family, and a multidisciplinary medical services group.

CHAPTER 3

Pediatric Renal Transplantation

Pediatric renal transplantation addresses a groundbreaking and life-saving intercession for youngsters with end-stage renal infection (ESRD) or serious kidney brokenness. This complex and multidisciplinary field of pediatric nephrology includes the careful transplantation of a sound kidney into a kid, either from a living benefactor, regularly a relative, or a departed giver. This investigation will dig into the complexities of pediatric renal transplantation, incorporating its signs, the transfer interaction, immunosuppressive treatments, long haul contemplations, and the significant effect on the existences of kids and their families.

1. **Signs for Pediatric Renal Transplantation:**
   Pediatric renal transplantation is looked at when as a kid encounters irreversible kidney disappointment, frequently coming about because of inborn irregularities, genetic kidney sicknesses, obtained problems, or confusions from a past kidney relocate. Normal signs incorporate innate oddities of the kidney and urinary parcel (CAKUT), inherited conditions, for example, polycystic kidney illness (PKD), and immune system or incendiary issues influencing the kidneys. Youngsters with end-stage renal sickness face huge difficulties in development, improvement, and by and large prosperity, making renal transplantation a basic mediation to reestablish kidney capability and upgrade their personal satisfaction.

2. **Assessment and Determination of Beneficiaries and Contributors:**
   The assessment and determination process for the two beneficiaries and living contributors is a careful and complete endeavor. Pediatric nephrologists, relocate specialists, and a multidisciplinary group survey the kid's general wellbeing, the seriousness of kidney brokenness, and any fundamental ailments. On account of living benefactors, the interaction includes a careful evaluation of the possible giver's physical and

mental wellbeing to guarantee that the contributor beneficiary match is reasonable and safe. Similarity factors, including blood classification and tissue coordinating, are basic contemplations in choosing contributors and limiting the gamble of dismissal.

3. **Surgery:**
The surgery for pediatric renal transplantation includes the fastidious expulsion of the solid kidney from the contributor and its transplantation into the beneficiary. In living giver transplantation, headways in careful strategies consider negligibly obtrusive systems, for example, laparoscopic contributor nephrectomy, which lessens recuperation time for the benefactor. For the beneficiary, the transfer system commonly includes setting the new kidney in the lower mid-region and associating its veins and ureter to the beneficiary's veins and bladder. Close coordination between the transfer careful group and pediatric sedation is critical to guarantee the security and outcome of the methodology.

4. **Immunosuppressive Treatments:**
Immunosuppressive treatments are a foundation of pediatric renal transplantation, pointed toward keeping the beneficiary's invulnerable framework from dismissing the relocated kidney. These meds, including calcineurin inhibitors, antimetabolites, and corticosteroids, are started not long from now previously or following transplantation. The measurements and mix of immunosuppressive medications are custom fitted to the youngster's particular requirements, determined to accomplish a fragile harmony between forestalling dismissal and limiting secondary effects. The deep rooted organization of these meds requires cautious observing for likely confusions, like contaminations, metabolic changes, and long haul consequences for bone wellbeing.

5. **Post-Relocate Checking and Care:**
The post-relocate period includes concentrated observing and mind to guarantee the progress of the transplantation and the general prosperity of the youngster. Close development with pediatric nephrologists, relocate specialists, and a multidisciplinary group is fundamental to evaluate kidney capability, oversee immunosuppressive prescriptions, and address any arising issues. Routine observing incorporates blood tests to evaluate kidney capability, helpful medication checking to advance immunosuppressive treatment, and imaging review to distinguish any underlying irregularities or intricacies. Long haul post-relocate care additionally includes tending to the psychosocial parts of transplantation, like the youngster's acclimation to the new kidney and the effect on the relational peculiarities.

6. **Confusions and Difficulties:**
Pediatric renal transplantation isn't without its intricacies and difficulties.

Dismissal, either intense or persistent, stays a critical worry regardless of advances in immunosuppressive treatments. The youngster's safe framework might perceive the relocated kidney as unfamiliar and mount an invulnerable reaction, prompting harm and expected loss of the unite. Diseases, especially in the underlying months after transplantation when immunosuppression is generally serious, represent an uplifted gamble. Furthermore, intricacies, for example, hypertension, post-relocate lymphoproliferative confusion (PTLD), and metabolic issues should be carefully checked and made due. The test lies in adjusting the requirement for immunosuppression to forestall dismissal with the gamble of complexities related with long haul immunosuppressive treatment.

7. **Development and Advancement Contemplations:**
Pediatric renal transplantation significantly impacts the development and advancement of beneficiaries. Youngsters with kidney disappointment frequently experience development impediment, postponed adolescence, and formative difficulties. Fruitful transplantation considers the reclamation of typical kidney capability, prompting enhancements in development, advancement, and by and large personal satisfaction. Be that as it may, the effect on development might shift, and a few youngsters might require extra intercessions or development chemical treatment to streamline their development potential.

8. **Psychosocial and Personal satisfaction Effect:**
The psychosocial parts of pediatric renal transplantation are foremost and stretch out past the clinical complexities of the method. The transfer venture includes huge changes for the kid and their family, enveloping close to home, social, and monetary aspects. The kid's transformation to the new kidney, adherence to medicine regimens, and the family's survival strategies all add to the psychosocial effect of transplantation. The help of pediatric analysts, social specialists, and care groups is basic in tending to the profound prosperity of both the youngster and their loved ones. Notwithstanding the difficulties, fruitful transplantation frequently brings about a significant improvement in the kid's personal satisfaction, permitting them to take part in typical youth exercises and seek after their instructive and social objectives.

9. **Long haul Results and Follow-Up:**
Long haul results in pediatric renal transplantation are dependent upon continuous checking, adherence to clinical regimens, and resolving arising issues. Effective transplantation can give fantastic kidney capability to numerous years, permitting beneficiaries to lead satisfying lives. Nonetheless, difficulties like ongoing dismissal, diseases, and the possible requirement for re-transplantation might emerge. The progress from pediatric to grown-up care represents one more basic point, requiring

consistent coordination to guarantee congruity of care and continuous help for the youthful grown-up beneficiary.

10. **Headways and Exploration in Pediatric Renal Transplantation:**
Headways and progressing research in pediatric renal transplantation add to further developed results and imaginative methodologies. Endeavors to refine immunosuppressive regimens, upgrade organ safeguarding strategies, and investigate options in contrast to customary immunosuppression hold guarantee for additional advancing the progress of pediatric renal transplantation. The reconciliation of accuracy medication, including genomics and biomarker research, may make ready for customized ways to deal with immunosuppression, decreasing the gamble of confusions and working on long haul results.

11. **Moral Contemplations and Benefactor Backing:**
The moral contemplations encompassing pediatric renal transplantation envelop issues connected with informed assent, contributor independence, and the cautious harmony between the advantages and dangers of transplantation. Support for living contributors, particularly when guardians or relatives act as benefactors, includes a careful comprehension of the expected effect on the giver's wellbeing and prosperity. Guaranteeing that contributors are completely educated, upheld, and get exhaustive post-gift care is fundamental in maintaining moral guidelines in pediatric renal transplantation.

12. **Worldwide Viewpoints and Admittance to Pediatric Renal Transplantation:**

Admittance to pediatric renal transplantation isn't uniform universally, featuring differences in medical care assets and framework. While pediatric transplantation is deeply grounded in some top level salary nations, obstructions to get to persevere in lower-pay areas. Addressing these variations includes endeavors to upgrade organ gift framework, grow relocate programs, and give schooling and assets to medical services experts in areas with restricted admittance. Cooperative drives at the worldwide level plan to work on the value and accessibility of pediatric renal transplantation for youngsters around the world.

3.1 Overview of Pediatric Renal Transplants

Pediatric renal transplantation remains as a momentous and life changing clinical mediation, offering youngsters with end-stage renal illness (ESRD) an opportunity at reestablished wellbeing and worked on personal satisfaction. This extensive outline will dive into the critical parts of pediatric renal transfers, including the signs for transplantation, the complicated course of organ acquisition and transplantation, postoperative consideration, immunosuppressive systems, long haul contemplations, and the significant effect on the existences of youngsters and their families.

1. **Signs for Pediatric Renal Transplantation:**
   Pediatric renal transplantation is looked at when as a kid's kidneys are practically compromised to the degree of end-stage renal illness (ESRD) or extreme brokenness, where moderate administration or dialysis is presently not a manageable choice.
   Signs for transplantation envelop an expansive range of conditions, including inherent oddities of the kidney and urinary parcel (CAKUT), inherited kidney sicknesses like polycystic kidney infection (PKD), glomerular problems, for example, central segmental glomerulosclerosis (FSGS), and obtained conditions like nephrotic disorder or immune system nephritis. The choice to seek after transplantation depends on an intensive evaluation of the youngster's general wellbeing, the seriousness of kidney brokenness, and the potential for further developed results with transplantation.

2. **Assessment and Choice of Beneficiaries:**
   The most common way of assessing and choosing beneficiaries for pediatric renal transplantation includes a multidisciplinary group of medical care experts, including pediatric nephrologists, relocate specialists, medical attendants, clinicians, and social laborers. The kid's clinical history, current wellbeing status, and any basic ailments are painstakingly surveyed to guarantee that transplantation is a feasible and useful choice. Pre-relocate assessments incorporate immunological appraisals, imaging studies to assess the urinary plot, and psychosocial evaluations to measure the kid's and family's status for transplantation. The objective is to recognize competitors who are probably going to profit from transplantation while limiting dangers and improving long haul results.

3. **Living Benefactor versus Perished Giver Transfers:**
   Pediatric renal transfers can be classified into living giver and expired contributor transfers. Living giver transfers include the careful expulsion of a kidney from a living benefactor, regularly a relative, and its transplantation into the beneficiary. Living giver transfers offer benefits like better organ quality, more limited holding up times, and the potential for precautionary transplantation before the youngster requires dialysis. Expired contributor transfers include the acquisition of kidneys from perished people, frequently through organ gift programs. The decision among living and expired contributor transplantation relies upon different elements, including the accessibility of appropriate benefactors, the kid's ailment, and the criticalness of transplantation.

4. **Surgery:**
   The surgery for pediatric renal transplantation is a perplexing and care-ful interaction that requires coordination between relocate specialists, pediatric anesthesiologists, and the transfer group. In living contributor transfers, high level careful strategies, for example, laparoscopic giver nephrectomy, might be utilized to limit the effect on the contributor's recuperation. The careful group cautiously puts the gave kidney in the lower mid-region of the beneficiary and associates its veins to the bene-ficiary's veins, guaranteeing legitimate blood stream. The ureter of the relocated kidney is then connected to the beneficiary's bladder. The out-come of the surgery establishes the groundwork for the resulting periods of postoperative consideration and long haul the board.

5. **Immunosuppressive Treatments:**
   Immunosuppressive treatments are a crucial part of pediatric renal trans-plantation, planning to keep the beneficiary's resistant framework from perceiving and dismissing the relocated kidney. These prescriptions, in-cluding calcineurin inhibitors, (for example, tacrolimus or cyclosporine), antimetabolites, (for example, mycophenolate mofetil or azathioprine), and corticosteroids, are started preceding or after transplantation. The decision and blend of immunosuppressive medications are custom-made to the kid's particular requirements, considering variables like age, weight, and expected aftereffects. The sensitive harmony between fore-stalling dismissal and limiting the gamble of irresistible complexities, metabolic changes, and opposite incidental effects requires progressing checking and acclimations to the immunosuppressive routine.

6. **Post-Relocate Checking and Care:**
   The post-relocate period is described by concentrated checking and mind to guarantee the outcome of the transplantation and the prosperity of the youngster. Standard subsequent encounters with the pediatric nephrol-ogy and relocate group are fundamental for evaluating kidney capability, overseeing immunosuppressive drugs, and resolving any arising issues. Blood tests, including appraisals of kidney capability and restorative med-ication observing of immunosuppressive meds, are regularly performed. Imaging studies, like ultrasounds, might be directed to assess the con-struction and capability of the relocated kidney. Close observing reaches out to the psychosocial parts of transplantation, tending to the kid's personal prosperity, school reintegration, and the effect on relational intricacies.

7. **Difficulties and Difficulties:**
   Pediatric renal transplantation isn't without its difficulties and ex-pected intricacies. Dismissal, either intense or persistent, stays a critical worry regardless of headways in immunosuppressive treatments. Intense

dismissal might happen soon after transplantation, requiring brief intercession with expanded immunosuppression. Constant dismissal, which can appear after some time, represents a continuous gamble to the drawn out progress of the transfer. Contaminations, particularly in the early post-relocate period when immunosuppression is generally extreme, address another huge test. Also, metabolic inconveniences, hypertension, and post-relocate lymphoproliferative confusion (PTLD) require watchful observing and the executives. Finding some kind of harmony between forestalling dismissal and limiting the gamble of difficulties is an unpredictable part of pediatric renal transplantation.

8. **Psychosocial and Personal satisfaction Effect:**
The psychosocial effect of pediatric renal transplantation is significant and envelops different aspects, including the kid's acclimation to the new kidney, the family's survival strategies, and the general effect on personal satisfaction. Pediatric clinicians and social laborers assume a vital part in supporting the profound prosperity of both the youngster and their family all through the transfer venture.

Instructive help guarantees a smooth progress back to school, addressing any likely interruptions because of the transfer cycle. The effective transplantation of a sound kidney frequently prompts a critical improvement in the youngster's personal satisfaction, permitting them to participate in typical youth exercises and seek after their instructive and social objectives.

9. **Long haul Results and Follow-Up:**
Long haul results in pediatric renal transplantation are dependent upon continuous checking, adherence to clinical regimens, and resolving arising issues. Effective transplantation can give great kidney capability to numerous years, permitting beneficiaries to lead satisfying lives. Be that as it may, difficulties like constant dismissal, diseases, and the expected requirement for re-transplantation might emerge. The change from pediatric to grown-up care represents one more basic crossroads, requiring consistent coordination to guarantee congruity of care and progressing support for the youthful grown-up beneficiary. Long haul follow-up includes checking kidney capability, overseeing immunosuppressive prescriptions, and addressing any arising inconveniences to safeguard the wellbeing and life span of the relocated kidney.

10. **Headways and Exploration in Pediatric Renal Transplantation:**
Progressing exploration and headways in pediatric renal transplantation add to further developed results and creative methodologies. Endeavors to refine immunosuppressive regimens, upgrade organ protection strategies, and investigate options in contrast to conventional immunosuppression hold guarantee for additional improving the progress of pediatric

renal transplantation. The joining of accuracy medication, including genomics and biomarker research, may make ready for customized ways to deal with immunosuppression, decreasing the gamble of entanglements and working on long haul results.

11. **Moral Contemplations and Giver Backing:**
    Moral contemplations assume a critical part in pediatric renal transplantation, especially in regards to informed assent, giver independence, and the cautious harmony between the advantages and dangers of transplantation. Support for living givers, particularly when guardians or relatives act as contributors, includes an exhaustive comprehension of the possible effect on the benefactor's wellbeing and prosperity. Guaranteeing that benefactors are completely educated, upheld, and get thorough post-gift care is fundamental in maintaining moral norms in pediatric renal transplantation.

12. **Worldwide Viewpoints and Admittance to Pediatric Renal Transplantation:**

Admittance to pediatric renal transplantation isn't uniform all around the world, highlighting abberations in medical care assets and foundation. While pediatric transplantation is deep rooted in some big league salary nations, obstructions to get to persevere in lower-pay districts.

Addressing these differences includes endeavors to improve organ gift framework, extend relocate programs, and give schooling and assets to medical services experts in locales with restricted admittance. Cooperative drives at the worldwide level plan to work on the value and accessibility of pediatric renal transplantation for kids around the world.

3.2 Challenges in Finding Suitable Donors

The mission for reasonable benefactors in pediatric renal transplantation is a mind boggling and multi-layered challenge that fundamentally impacts the achievement and accessibility of life-saving kidney transfers for youngsters confronting end-stage renal illness (ESRD) or serious kidney brokenness. This investigation will dig into the bunch difficulties experienced in tracking down appropriate contributors for pediatric renal transplantation, enveloping viewpoints like benefactor similarity, moral contemplations, living giver elements, expired contributor accessibility, and the worldwide variations in admittance to transplantation.

1. **Contributor Similarity and Immunological Difficulties:**
   One of the essential difficulties in finding reasonable contributors for pediatric renal transplantation lies in accomplishing similarity between the benefactor and beneficiary. Immunological similarity is essential to

limit the gamble of dismissal, a cycle where the beneficiary's insusceptible framework perceives the relocated kidney as unfamiliar and mounts a safe reaction. Matching blood classifications and leading intensive immunological evaluations, including human leukocyte antigen (HLA) composing, are fundamental parts of the benefactor beneficiary matching interaction. The shortage of impeccably paired benefactors inside families or everyone represents a critical test, frequently requiring cautious thought of elective methodologies and immunosuppressive techniques to relieve the gamble of dismissal.

2. **Living Giver Elements and Moral Contemplations:**
   Living givers, commonly relatives, assume a urgent part in pediatric renal transplantation, offering the potential for ideal and precautionary transplantation. In any case, exploring the elements of living benefactor connections presents moral contemplations and difficulties. The choice for a relative to act as a living benefactor includes cautious assessment of the likely effect on the giver's wellbeing, both present moment and long haul. Adjusting the charitable longing to save the existence of a friend or family member with the moral basic to defend the prosperity of the living benefactor requires exhaustive instruction, directing, and moral oversight. Guaranteeing informed assent, safeguarding benefactor independence, and tending to the psychosocial parts of living gift are fundamental parts in the moral structure encompassing living contributor transplantation.

3. **Psychosocial and Monetary Contemplations for Living Benefactors:**
   The difficulties in finding reasonable benefactors stretch out past clinical contemplations to envelop psychosocial and monetary aspects, especially for living givers.
   The choice to give a kidney includes the likely actual dangers as well as contemplations connected with the benefactor's personal prosperity, personal satisfaction, and monetary steadiness. Living givers might confront difficulties like the effect on business, expected changes in insurability, and the drawn out mental impacts of gift. Moral and psychosocial support for living givers is indispensable to tending to these contemplations, guaranteeing that the choice to give is made with full mindfulness and backing.

4. **Expired Giver Accessibility and Organ Deficiency:**
   The accessibility of expired givers is a basic variable impacting the admittance to kidney transplantation for pediatric patients. The interest for kidney transfers far surpasses the stock of organs from perished givers, prompting a steady organ deficiency. Youngsters might confront extra difficulties in getting to expired contributor kidneys because of the prioritization of grown-up beneficiaries and the allotment approaches set up. The restricted pool of expired benefactors highlights the direness

of augmenting living contributor choices and pushing for strategies that focus on evenhanded access for pediatric patients.

5. **Designation Approaches and Pediatric Prioritization:** Designation strategies inside organ obtainment associations and transplantation networks assume a critical part in figuring out which patients get accessible organs. Challenges emerge in adjusting the critical requirement for pediatric transfers with the standards of reasonableness and value in organ designation. The prioritization of pediatric beneficiaries is a nuanced thought, as it includes gauging the potential for worked on long haul results in youngsters against the prompt direness of relocating organs into grown-up beneficiaries. Backing for strategies that address the novel necessities of pediatric patients and guarantee fair admittance to perished contributor kidneys is a continuous test in the field of pediatric renal transplantation.

6. **Worldwide Abberations in Admittance to Transplantation:** The difficulties in finding reasonable benefactors are additionally exacerbated by worldwide differences in admittance to pediatric renal transplantation. While transplantation is deeply grounded in major league salary nations with strong medical services foundations, lower-pay locales might confront hindrances connected with organ gift framework, medical services assets, and monetary imperatives. Abberations in access add to unjust results for youngsters in areas with restricted transplantation abilities. Addressing these worldwide abberations includes cooperative endeavors to improve organ gift rehearses, grow relocate programs, and give schooling and assets to medical care experts in underserved locales.

7. **Public Mindfulness and Organ Gift Rates:** Public mindfulness about the significance of organ gift, especially with regards to pediatric transplantation, stays a critical test. Numerous areas battle with low organ gift rates because of elements like absence of mindfulness, social convictions, and worries about the organ gift process.
Drives to teach the general population, scatter legends encompassing organ gift, and encourage a culture of selflessness are vital in tending to this test. Further developing organ gift rates benefits pediatric beneficiaries as well as improves the general achievement and accessibility of transplantation for people, everything being equal.

8. **Clinical and Psychosocial Assessment of Expected Contributors:** Directing exhaustive clinical and psychosocial assessments of potential benefactors presents its own arrangement of difficulties. Guaranteeing the contributor's physical and mental readiness for gift requires extensive appraisals, including cardiovascular and renal assessments, as well as mental screenings. The objective is to limit dangers to the benefactor while defending their prosperity. Nonetheless, difficulties might emerge

in situations where potential contributors have previous ailments, raising moral problems about the appropriateness of gift and the expected effect on the giver's drawn out wellbeing.

9. **Legitimate and Moral Structures for Organ Gift:**
   Legitimate and moral systems encompassing organ gift fluctuate all around the world and inside various purviews. Laying out clear and moral rules for organ gift, especially with regards to living benefactors, is fundamental to safeguard the freedoms and prosperity of all gatherings included. Guaranteeing consistence with laid out moral principles, informed assent systems, and legitimate insurances for contributors is a continuous test that requires joint effort between medical services experts, lawful specialists, and ethicists.

10. **Advancements in Giver Choice and Acquisition:**
    Headways in clinical innovation and developments in giver choice and obtainment address a promising road for tending to the difficulties in tracking down reasonable contributors. Strategies, for example, laparoscopic giver nephrectomy have limited the intrusiveness of living contributor techniques, decreasing recuperation times and likely difficulties. Continuous investigation into novel methodologies, including matched kidney trade programs and high level imaging advancements, expects to grow the pool of appropriate benefactors and enhance matching systems for pediatric beneficiaries.

11. **Social and Strict Points of view on Organ Gift:**
    Social and strict convictions encompassing organ gift can essentially affect the eagerness of people and families to partake in organ gift. Difficulties might emerge in situations where social or strict convictions struggle with the standards of organ transplantation. Aversion to social variety and deferential commitment with assorted networks are fundamental in tending to these difficulties, encouraging open exchange, and advancing comprehension about the life-saving capability of organ gift.

12. **Mechanical Advances in Organ Safeguarding:**

The difficulties in finding appropriate givers additionally stretch out to the protection of given organs before transplantation. Mechanical advances in organ conservation, including machine perfusion and hypothermic stockpiling procedures, plan to improve the suitability and nature of giver kidneys. Enhancing organ conservation advancements is basic for growing the geographic reach of organ obtainment and improving the probability of fruitful transfer results.

3.3 Triumphs in Successful Transplant Cases

Wins in fruitful pediatric renal transfer cases reverberate with the ground-breaking force of clinical progressions, devoted medical services groups, and the versatility of youngsters confronting end-stage renal illness (ESRD) or serious kidney brokenness. These victories address the reclamation of kidney capability as well as the unfurling of stories set apart by trust, versatility, and the quest for a more promising time to come. In investigating the victories in effective pediatric renal transfer cases, we dig into the significant effect on the existences of beneficiaries, the cooperative endeavors of medical services experts, and the persistent advancement of transplantation rehearses.

1. **Reclamation of Kidney Capability and Worked on Personal satisfaction:**
   The essential victory in effective pediatric renal transfer cases lies in the reclamation of kidney capability, freeing youngsters from the imperatives of dialysis and the difficulties presented by compromised renal wellbeing. Following a fruitful transfer, beneficiaries experience a critical improvement in their general prosperity and personal satisfaction. Liberated from the requirements of persistent kidney illness, youngsters can take part in ordinary youth exercises, go to class routinely, and partake in sports and social cooperations, denoting a victory over the impediments forced by ESRD.

2. **Preplanned Transfers and Aversion of Dialysis:**
   Wins in pediatric renal transplantation reach out to situations where pre-planned transfers are accomplished, permitting beneficiaries to sidestep the requirement for dialysis through and through. Precautionary transplantation, performed before the beginning of dialysis, offers various benefits, including better long haul join endurance and worked on generally speaking results. The evasion of dialysis addresses a critical victory, saving kids from the physical and mental weights related with delayed dialysis medicines.

3. **Living Giver Examples of overcoming adversity and Family Strength:**
   Many victories in pediatric renal transplantation revolve around living benefactor examples of overcoming adversity, especially when relatives step forward as benevolent givers. These accounts represent the strength and fortitude inside families, where guardians, kin, or more distant family individuals become residing benefactors to save the existence of a kid.
   The victory reaches out past the clinical progress of the transfer to the significant effect on relational peculiarities, encouraging a feeling of solidarity, common perspective, and the festival of life.

4. **Long haul Achievement and Unite Endurance:**
   Long haul achievement and supported unite endurance address wins in pediatric renal transplantation, underscoring the strength of the relocated

kidney and its capacity to give proceeded with kidney capability throughout the long term. Youngsters who experience long haul accomplishment after transplantation frequently develop into adulthood with their relocated kidneys, accomplishing achievements, seeking after instruction and vocations, and driving satisfying lives. The victory of supported unite endurance highlights the progressions in immunosuppressive treatments, organ protection procedures, and post-relocate care.

5. **Headways in Immunotherapy and Dismissal Counteraction:**
Wins in pediatric renal transplantation are intently attached to headways in immunotherapy and dismissal counteraction. The capacity to regulate the resistant reaction actually has added to diminished paces of intense and constant dismissal, working on the general progress of relocate techniques. Fitting immunosuppressive regimens to individual patient profiles and limiting the gamble of confusions address wins in the field, permitting kids to profit from the life-saving capability of transplantation without undermining their drawn out wellbeing.

6. **Accuracy Medication and Customized Treatment Approaches:**
The rise of accuracy medication in pediatric renal transplantation addresses a victory in fitting treatment ways to deal with the exceptional hereditary and sub-atomic profiles of individual patients. The capacity to recognize explicit hereditary markers, survey the gamble of dismissal, and customize immunosuppressive regimens adds to advanced results. Accuracy medication holds guarantee for additional upgrading the progress of pediatric renal transplantation and limiting unfavorable impacts, denoting a victory in the period of customized and designated treatments.

7. **Effective Transfers in Sharpened Beneficiaries:**
Wins in pediatric renal transplantation reach out to situations where sharpened beneficiaries, with prior antibodies that increment the gamble of dismissal, go through fruitful transfers. Beating the difficulties presented by refinement requires creative methodologies, including desensitization conventions and high level immunological matching procedures. Effective transfers in sharpened beneficiaries feature the strength of medical care groups in exploring complex immunological scenes and giving life-saving open doors to youngsters who could confront elevated hindrances to transplantation.

8. **Developments in Organ Protection and Relocate Methods:**
Developments in organ protection methods and relocate methodology add to the victories in effective pediatric renal transfer cases. Machine perfusion, hypothermic capacity, and refined careful methods upgrade the suitability and nature of relocated kidneys. These progressions bring about superior join capability, diminished ischemia-reperfusion injury,

and expanded open doors for effective transplantation, stamping wins at the convergence of clinical innovation and careful advancement.

9. **Psychosocial Backing and Effective Changes:**
The victories in pediatric renal transplantation stretch out past clinical results to envelop psychosocial support and fruitful changes for beneficiaries. The arrangement of far reaching psychosocial support, including advising, instructive help, and help with school reintegration, adds to the general prosperity of relocate beneficiaries. Fruitful changes from pediatric to grown-up care address wins in coherence of care, guaranteeing progressing backing and observing for youthful grown-ups who have gone through effective renal transfers.

10. **Worldwide Joint efforts and Worldwide Examples of overcoming adversity:**
Wins in pediatric renal transplantation manifest on a worldwide scale through global joint efforts and examples of overcoming adversity. Shared ability, cooperative examination attempts, and the trading of best practices add to further developed results for kids around the world. Worldwide examples of overcoming adversity feature the limit of medical services frameworks to defeat geological obstructions, address variations in access, and proposition life-saving open doors to youngsters confronting renal difficulties, checking wins chasing after worldwide wellbeing value.

11. **Backing and Expanded Mindfulness:**
Wins in pediatric renal transplantation are additionally moved by support endeavors and expanded mindfulness about the significance of organ gift. Effective transfer cases frequently act as impetuses for uplifted mindfulness, motivating networks to participate in conversations about organ gift, disperse fantasies, and encourage a culture of selflessness. The victories in promotion add to the development of organ gift vaults, expanded public help, and a better climate for working with effective pediatric renal transfers.

12. **Patient and Family Strengthening:**

The strengthening of relocate beneficiaries and their families addresses a victory in the comprehensive way to deal with pediatric renal transplantation. Giving schooling, assets, and backing to patients and their families engages them to effectively take part in the administration of post-relocate care. Wins in persistent and family strengthening add to better adherence to clinical regimens, further developed correspondence with medical care suppliers, and upgraded generally speaking prosperity.

CHAPTER 4

Hemodialysis and Peritoneal Dialysis in Children

Hemodialysis and peritoneal dialysis stand as life-supporting treatments for youngsters confronting end-stage renal illness (ESRD) or extreme kidney brokenness, giving a scaffold to renal transplantation or, at times, filling in as a drawn out renal substitution treatment. This far reaching investigation dives into the subtleties of hemodialysis and peritoneal dialysis in kids, enveloping their standards, signs, benefits, challenges, and the effect on the existences of youthful patients and their families.

1. **Standards of Hemodialysis in Kids:**
   Hemodialysis is a renal substitution treatment that includes the extracorporeal expulsion of poisons and overabundance liquids from the blood. In youngsters, hemodialysis is commonly performed utilizing particular hardware intended to oblige the novel requirements and sizes of pediatric patients.
   The cycle includes the situation of a vascular access, normally a focal venous catheter or an arteriovenous fistula, to permit the blood to be removed, purged through a dialyzer, and afterward got back to the kid's course. Hemodialysis depends on the standards of dissemination and ultrafiltration to accomplish solute and liquid evacuation, impersonating the physiological elements of the kidneys.
2. **Signs for Hemodialysis in Pediatric Patients:**
   Hemodialysis turns into a need for pediatric patients when their kidneys are presently not ready to really carry out the significant roles of separating side-effects and keeping up with liquid and electrolyte balance. Normal signs for hemodialysis in youngsters incorporate end-stage renal illness, intense kidney injury, serious electrolyte irregular characteristics, and liquid over-burden. In intense settings, hemodialysis might act as a brief mediation to balance out the youngster's condition, while in

instances of constant kidney sickness, it very well may be a drawn out restorative methodology until renal transplantation becomes doable.

3. **Vascular Access in Pediatric Hemodialysis:**
Vascular access is a basic part of hemodialysis in kids, as it straight-forwardly influences the effectiveness and wellbeing of the strategy. Pediatric patients might have exceptional difficulties as far as vascular access because of their more modest size and explicit physical contemplations. Focal venous catheters, arteriovenous fistulas, and arteriovenous unions are among the normally used admittance choices in pediatric hemodialysis. The decision of vascular access relies upon elements like the kid's age, vascular life systems, expected span of dialysis, and the requirement for sure fire access in intense circumstances.

4. **Benefits of Hemodialysis in Kids:**
Hemodialysis offers a few benefits in the administration of pediatric renal substitution treatment. One huge benefit is the fast evacuation of poisons and abundance liquids, making it especially powerful in intense circumstances like extreme electrolyte irregular characteristics or liquid over-burden. Hemodialysis is likewise helpful for discontinuous planning, permitting youngsters to keep a more adaptable way of life between dialysis meetings. Moreover, the unified idea of hemodialysis units gives a steady climate where particular pediatric nephrology and dialysis groups can intently screen and address the particular necessities of youthful patients.

5. **Difficulties of Hemodialysis in Pediatric Settings:**
While hemodialysis is a vital remedial methodology, it accompanies its arrangement of difficulties, especially in pediatric settings. Vascular access-related intricacies, like contaminations and apoplexy, can present critical dangers to pediatric patients. The requirement for anticoagulation during hemodialysis adds intricacy, requiring cautious administration to forestall draining complexities. In addition, the need for customary visits to hemodialysis units might disturb the day to day schedules of pediatric patients and their families, affecting school participation, social exercises, and by and large personal satisfaction.

6. **Peritoneal Dialysis: Standards and Methods:**
Peritoneal dialysis is an option renal substitution treatment that uses the peritoneal layer as a characteristic semipermeable channel. In kids, peritoneal dialysis is frequently liked because of its relative effortlessness, lower specialized requests, and potential for locally situated administration. The cycle includes the instillation of a dialysis arrangement into the peritoneal hole through a catheter. The peritoneal film takes into consideration the dissemination and ultrafiltration of side-effects and

overabundance liquids, and after a stay time, the spent dialysis arrangement is depleted, finishing one pattern of peritoneal dialysis.

7. **Signs for Peritoneal Dialysis in Pediatric Patients:**
Peritoneal dialysis is demonstrated in various pediatric renal circumstances, including ongoing kidney illness, end-stage renal sickness, and intense kidney injury. It is a reasonable choice for kids anticipating renal transplantation or the people who may not be prompt contender for transplantation. Peritoneal dialysis is especially beneficial in babies and small kids, offering a gentler and more nonstop type of dialysis that lines up with their physiological requirements.

8. **Catheter Situation and Strategies in Pediatric Peritoneal Dialysis:**
The progress of peritoneal dialysis in youngsters depends on the appropriate situation and care of the peritoneal dialysis catheter. The catheter is normally embedded into the peritoneal cavity through a surgery, and its legitimate situating is significant for viable dialysis. Pediatric patients might go through catheter situation under broad sedation, and the determination of catheter type (Tenckhoff, swan neck, and so on) relies upon the kid's age and size. Cautious thoughtfulness regarding aseptic strategy during catheter situation limits the gamble of disease, a typical worry in peritoneal dialysis.

9. **Benefits of Peritoneal Dialysis in Kids:**
Peritoneal dialysis offers particular benefits in the pediatric populace. One of the key advantages is the potential for locally established treatment, permitting families to oversee peritoneal dialysis in the solace of their homes. This not just limits the disturbance to the kid's regular routine yet in addition engages families to partake being taken care of by their kid effectively. The constant idea of peritoneal dialysis gives a more physiological methodology, keeping a more steady interior climate contrasted with the irregular idea of hemodialysis.

10. **Difficulties of Peritoneal Dialysis in Pediatric Settings:**
In spite of its benefits, peritoneal dialysis presents difficulties in pediatric settings. Contamination, especially peritonitis, is a huge concern, underlining the significance of careful sterile methods during trades. Kids may likewise confront difficulties connected with liquid equilibrium, as the nonstop idea of peritoneal dialysis might affect the retention of liquids from the dialysate, requiring changes in the treatment plan. Moreover, worries about catheter-related complexities, including impediment or spillage, require cautious checking and opportune mediations.

11. **Effect on the Existences of Pediatric Patients and Families:**
Both hemodialysis and peritoneal dialysis significantly affect the existences of pediatric patients and their families. The requirement for standard dialysis meetings, whether in a hemodialysis unit or at home

for peritoneal dialysis, acquaints huge changes with everyday schedules. Youngsters on dialysis might confront limitations in diet and liquid admission, affecting their social connections and cooperation in exercises. Families assume a urgent part in offering profound help, overseeing dialysis plans, and exploring the difficulties related with the picked methodology.

12. **Progress to Renal Transplantation:**
For the vast majority pediatric patients on dialysis, a definitive objective is many times renal transplantation, offering the commitment of reestablished kidney capability and a day to day existence liberated from continuous dialysis meetings. Both hemodialysis and peritoneal dialysis act as imperative crossing over treatments, supporting youngsters while they anticipate transplantation. The effective progress from dialysis to transplantation addresses a victory in the excursion of pediatric patients, denoting the start of another part described by recharged wellbeing and worked on personal satisfaction.

13. **Constant Advancement and Exploration in Pediatric Dialysis:**

The field of pediatric dialysis keeps on advancing, driven by continuous exploration pointed toward improving treatments, upgrading results, and tending to the exceptional difficulties looked by youthful patients. Progresses in dialysis innovation, worked on comprehension of pediatric-explicit pharmacokinetics, and advancements in vascular access and catheter configuration add to the consistent development of pediatric dialysis rehearses. Research tries likewise investigate ways of moderating the drawn out entanglements related with dialysis, with an emphasis on limiting the effect on development, neurocognitive turn of events, and by and large prosperity.

4.1 Navigating Challenges in Pediatric Dialysis
Exploring the difficulties in pediatric dialysis addresses a mind boggling venture including medical services suppliers, youthful patients, and their families. The domain of pediatric dialysis, enveloping both hemodialysis and peritoneal dialysis, is laden with special obstructions that require cautious thought, transformation, and cooperative endeavors to guarantee ideal results. This investigation dives into the complex difficulties looked in pediatric dialysis, analyzing issues connected with vascular access, treatment adherence, psychosocial effect, development and advancement, and the all-encompassing objective of changing to renal transplantation.

1. **Vascular Access Difficulties:**
Vascular access is a basic part of pediatric dialysis, impacting the productivity and security of the methodology. Youngsters might confront

difficulties connected with the size and availability of their vasculature. Focal venous catheters, generally utilized for hemodialysis in pediatric patients, can be related with difficulties like diseases, apoplexy, and the requirement for regular substitutions. Exploring the intricacies of vascular access in pediatric dialysis includes a multidisciplinary approach, with cautious thought of the kid's age, life structures, and the expected span of dialysis. The test lies in adjusting the requirement for successful dialysis with limiting the dangers related with vascular access-related confusions.

2. **Adherence to Treatment Regimens:**
Guaranteeing adherence to dialysis treatment regimens represents a critical test in pediatric consideration. Kids going through dialysis frequently face disturbances to their day to day routines, remembering limitations for diet, liquid admission, and cooperation in exercises. The multifaceted harmony between the requests of dialysis and keeping a similarity to predictability in the existences of pediatric patients requires dynamic contribution from both the youngster and their loved ones. Non-adherence to treatment regimens can prompt confusions, poor dialysis results, and effect the general wellbeing and prosperity of the kid. Tending to this challenge includes cultivating a steady climate, giving training, and incorporating procedures to improve treatment adherence.

3. **Psychosocial Effect on Pediatric Patients:**
The psychosocial effect of pediatric dialysis reaches out past the physiological parts of the treatment. Youngsters going through dialysis might encounter profound trouble, tension, and interruptions to their social cooperations. The test lies in tending to the mental prosperity of pediatric patients, perceiving the possible effect on their emotional wellness and by and large personal satisfaction. Psychosocial support, including guiding administrations for both the kid and their family, assumes an essential part in exploring this test. Coordinating age-fitting mediations and including youngster life experts can add to establishing a positive and strong climate for pediatric patients going through dialysis.

4. **Influence on Development and Advancement:**
Pediatric patients on dialysis face difficulties connected with development and advancement. Ongoing kidney sickness, intensified by the impacts of dialysis, can influence straight development, bone wellbeing, and in general turn of events. The test is to moderate these impacts through cautious observing, wholesome intercessions, and development chemical treatment when shown. Adjusting the wholesome necessities of developing kids with the dietary limitations forced by dialysis requires a nuanced approach. The cooperative endeavors of pediatric nephrologists, dietitians, and other unified medical care experts are essential in

exploring this test and improving the development and advancement of pediatric patients on dialysis.

5. **Progress to Renal Transplantation:**
A urgent objective in the excursion of pediatric patients on dialysis is the change to renal transplantation. While dialysis fills in as a daily existence supporting treatment, a definitive point is frequently to furnish youngsters with a renal transfer, offering the potential for reestablished kidney capability and a day to day existence liberated from progressing dialysis meetings. Exploring the pathway to transplantation includes tending to immunological difficulties, guaranteeing ideal pre-relocate the executives, and planning the mind boggling coordinated operations related with organ transplantation. The test lies in working with a consistent progress, limiting the span of dialysis while expanding the possibilities of an effective renal transfer. Coordination between dialysis groups, relocate groups, and progressing multidisciplinary care is fundamental in conquering this test.

6. **Instructive Difficulties for Pediatric Patients:**
Pediatric patients on dialysis might confront instructive difficulties because of the requests of their treatment regimens. Continuous dialysis meetings, clinical arrangements, and potential complexities can disturb standard school participation and effect scholastic execution. The test is to help the instructive requirements of pediatric patients, guaranteeing congruity in their scholastic interests. Coordinated effort between medical care suppliers, teachers, and school heads is essential in creating methodologies, for example, locally established learning, adaptable school timetables, and backing for scholarly facilities. Addressing instructive difficulties adds to the all encompassing consideration of pediatric patients on dialysis, cultivating their scholarly development close by their actual prosperity.

7. **Monetary and Financial Ramifications:**
The monetary and financial ramifications of pediatric dialysis add one more layer of intricacy to the difficulties looked by families. Dialysis includes significant medical services costs, including costs connected with prescriptions, vascular access upkeep, and expected hospitalizations. Families might experience difficulties connected with protection inclusion, personal costs, and the expected effect on parental work due to providing care liabilities. Social laborers and monetary guides assume a pivotal part in supporting families through these difficulties, exploring protection issues, getting to monetary help programs, and giving assets to moderate the financial weight related with pediatric dialysis.

8. **Disease Control and Entanglements:**
Disease control is a principal worry in pediatric dialysis, particularly for

those going through peritoneal dialysis. Peritonitis, an irritation of the peritoneal film, is a potential entanglement that can prompt huge bleakness. The test is to execute thorough contamination control works on, including fastidious aseptic strategies during catheter care and dialysate trades. Schooling of both medical services suppliers and families on perceiving early indications of contamination and brief mediation is fundamental in limiting the gamble of peritonitis. Hemodialysis, including vascular access, likewise conveys a gamble of access-related contaminations, requiring careful reconnaissance and preventive measures.

9. **Pediatric-Explicit Treatment Difficulties:**
Pediatric patients present exceptional provokes in dialysis because of their shifting sizes, formative stages, and physiological contrasts. Dosing drugs, overseeing liquid equilibrium, and changing dialysis boundaries require pediatric-explicit contemplations. The test is to fit dialysis medicines to the singular requirements of every kid, representing variables like age, weight, development direction, and formative achievements. Pediatric nephrologists, medical caretakers, and different individuals from the medical care group should team up near adjust therapy conventions and guarantee the wellbeing and viability of dialysis in the pediatric populace.

10. **Relational peculiarities and Guardian Stress:**
The difficulties in pediatric dialysis stretch out to the elements inside families and the pressure experienced via parental figures. The requests of dealing with a youngster on dialysis can be sincerely and truly burdening for guardians and other relatives. Parental figure pressure might influence the general relational intricacy, requiring procedures for adapting, versatility, and consistent reassurance. Pediatric nephrology groups assume an imperative part in perceiving and tending to parental figure pressure, giving assets to help, and encouraging open correspondence to explore the difficulties looked by groups of pediatric patients on dialysis.

11. **Challenges in Locally established Dialysis Care:**
For pediatric patients on peritoneal dialysis, locally established care presents its arrangement of difficulties. While locally established peritoneal dialysis offers the benefit of expanded adaptability and diminished disturbance to day to day existence, it requires extensive schooling and preparing for families. The test lies in engaging parental figures to perform dialysis trades, oversee gear, and perceive indications of possible complexities. Continuous help, ordinary correspondence with the medical care group, and admittance to assets, for example, telehealth administrations are fundamental in exploring the difficulties related with locally situated dialysis care for pediatric patients.

12. **Support for Pediatric Dialysis Patients:**

Tending to the difficulties in pediatric dialysis requires promotion at different levels, including neighborhood medical care frameworks, strategy making bodies, and the more extensive local area. Backing endeavors center around bringing issues to light about the interesting necessities of pediatric patients on dialysis, elevating exploration to further develop results, and affecting arrangements that help extensive pediatric nephrology care. Backing likewise stretches out to drives that cultivate a steady climate for families, address differences in admittance to mind, and elevate a comprehensive way to deal with the prosperity of pediatric patients going through dialysis.

4.2 Triumphs of Successful Dialysis Management

Wins in effective dialysis the board for pediatric patients embody the aggregate endeavors of medical services groups, families, and the versatility of youthful patients confronting end-stage renal sickness (ESRD) or extreme kidney brokenness. These victories length a range of accomplishments, from the streamlining of treatment modalities and relieving difficulties to the fulfillment of worked on personal satisfaction and fruitful changes to renal transplantation. Investigating the victories of fruitful dialysis the board reveals insight into the positive results, forward leaps, and progressions that shape the account of pediatric nephrology.

1. **Ideal Treatment Methodology Choice:**
   One of the early victories in fruitful dialysis the board is the prudent determination of the ideal treatment methodology for each pediatric patient. The cautious thought of variables like age, size, ailment, and way of life adds to the customized decision among hemodialysis and peritoneal dialysis. Fitting the treatment methodology to the singular necessities and conditions of the youngster addresses a victory that sets the establishment for compelling dialysis the board.

2. **Vascular Access Examples of overcoming adversity:**
   Wins in vascular access, critical for hemodialysis, manifest in examples of overcoming adversity of unhampered blood stream, limited contamination rates, and delayed admittance life span. Headways in vascular access methods and continuous advancements add to these victories, permitting pediatric patients to go through hemodialysis with diminished entanglements and worked on personal satisfaction. The accomplishment of solid vascular access denotes a critical victory in the general progress of dialysis the board.

3. **Upgraded Treatment Adherence and Patient Commitment:**
   Effective dialysis the board frequently includes wins in treatment adherence and patient commitment. Kids and their families assume a functioning part in sticking to therapy regimens, including dietary limitations, liquid admission impediments, and prescription timetables. Wins in this

viewpoint mirror the cooperation between medical services suppliers and families, encouraging a feeling of strengthening and obligation in pediatric patients. Schooling, continuous help, and open correspondence add to these victories, guaranteeing that youngsters effectively take part in their dialysis care.

4. **Psychosocial Prosperity and Steady Conditions:**
Wins in psychosocial prosperity highlight the significance of establishing steady conditions for pediatric patients going through dialysis. Psychosocial support drives, including directing administrations, kid life subject matter experts, and friend support programs, add to the close to home strength of youthful patients.

Wins in this space are apparent when kids on dialysis are genuinely supported as well as experience positive psychological wellness, social joining, and a superior in general personal satisfaction.

5. **Development and Improvement Achievements:**
Effective dialysis the board is set apart by wins in accomplishing development and formative achievements in pediatric patients. In spite of the difficulties presented by constant kidney sickness and dialysis, mediations like development chemical treatment, nourishing help, and cautious checking add to positive results. Wins in this domain manifest as pediatric patients accomplish age-fitting development, bone wellbeing, and formative advancement, mirroring the devotion of medical services groups to improve the general prosperity of youthful patients.

6. **Smooth Changes to Renal Transplantation:**
An essential victory in the excursion of pediatric patients on dialysis is the fruitful change to renal transplantation. This accomplishment addresses a shift from the limitations of progressing dialysis to the commitment of reestablished kidney capability and a daily existence freed from standard dialysis meetings. Wins in working with smooth advances include fastidious pre-relocate the executives, coordination among dialysis and relocate groups, and tending to immunological difficulties. Each fruitful renal transfer is a victory that denotes the start of another section for pediatric patients, offering recharged trust and worked on long haul results.

7. **Scholastic and Instructive Accomplishments:**
Wins in fruitful dialysis the board stretch out to scholarly and instructive accomplishments for pediatric patients. In spite of the disturbances brought about by dialysis medicines, pediatric patients can flourish scholastically with the backing of medical care groups, teachers, and school overseers. Adaptable instructive game plans, locally situated learning, and instructive promotion add to wins where pediatric patients on dialysis can seek after their scholarly objectives, encouraging a feeling of predictability and accomplishment.

8. **Moderation of Inconveniences and Contaminations:**
   The effective administration of pediatric dialysis includes wins in moderating entanglements and diseases. Careful observation, adherence to contamination control measures, and incite intercession add to wins where pediatric patients experience negligible confusions during dialysis. Propels in contamination avoidance procedures, catheter care conventions, and the utilization of antimicrobial specialists epitomize the victories accomplished in guaranteeing the security and prosperity of youthful patients going through dialysis.

9. **Strengthening of Parental figures and Families:**
   Wins in effective dialysis the board stretch out to the strengthening of guardians and families.
   The excursion of pediatric patients on dialysis frequently includes a co-operative exertion, with families assuming a significant part in day to day care, therapy adherence, and exploring the difficulties related with persistent kidney illness. Giving assets, schooling, and daily reassurance to parental figures addresses a victory in cultivating a strong and enabled emotionally supportive network for pediatric patients.

10. **Progressions in Pediatric Dialysis Innovation:**
    Wins in pediatric dialysis the board are entwined with progressions in innovation planned explicitly for the remarkable necessities of youthful patients. Advancements in pediatric dialysis machines, locally situated dialysis hardware, and wearable gadgets add to wins where treatment turns out to be more productive, open, and customized to the pediatric populace. Mechanical progressions upgrade the general dialysis experience for youngsters, lessening obstructions to treatment and working on their general personal satisfaction.

11. **Promotion for Pediatric Nephrology Care:**
    Wins in effective dialysis the board stretch out to backing endeavors that advance mindfulness, examination, and strategies supporting pediatric nephrology care. Backing drives mean to address variations in admittance to mind, impact medical care strategies, and cultivate an all encompassing way to deal with the prosperity of pediatric patients going through dialysis. Wins in backing add to the perceivability of pediatric nephrology on nearby, public, and worldwide stages, accentuating the significance of devoted care for youthful patients confronting renal difficulties.

12. **Flexibility and Positive Results in Pediatric Dialysis:**

A definitive victory in fruitful dialysis the board is the flexibility exhibited by pediatric patients and their families even with constant kidney sickness. Regardless of the difficulties, mishaps, and changes required, numerous youngsters on dialysis display momentous flexibility. Positive results, including further developed wellbeing, psychosocial prosperity, and fruitful advances to renal transplantation, encapsulate the victories of the cooperative endeavors of medical care suppliers, families, and the inherent strength of youthful patients.

4.3 Quality of Life Considerations

Personal satisfaction contemplations in the domain of pediatric nephrology, especially for youngsters going through dialysis or living with renal problems, comprise a multi-layered and essential part of care. The mind boggling balance between dealing with the actual parts of the illness, the psychosocial influence on the kid and their family, and the quest for a satisfying and significant life characterizes the scene of personal satisfaction in pediatric nephrology.

This investigation dives into the different elements of personal satisfaction contemplations, incorporating the effect of renal issues on day to day existence, mediations to improve prosperity, and the general objective of streamlining the general personal satisfaction for youthful patients confronting renal difficulties.

1. **Effect of Renal Issues on Day to day existence:**
   Renal issues, particularly those requiring dialysis or prompting persistent kidney illness (CKD), significantly affect the regular routines of pediatric patients. The thorough requests of dialysis regimens, dietary limitations, and liquid admission constraints can upset ordinary schedules and exercises. Youngsters confronting renal difficulties might encounter limits in their capacity to go to class consistently, take part in sports, and participate in friendly collaborations. The effect stretches out to the whole family, as guardians might have to explore complex therapy regimens, regular clinical arrangements, and possible hospitalizations. Understanding and addressing these difficulties are major to surveying and working on the general personal satisfaction for pediatric patients with renal issues.

2. **Actual Prosperity and Side effect The board:**
   Personal satisfaction contemplations in pediatric nephrology require an emphasis on the actual prosperity of youthful patients. Side effects related with renal issues, like exhaustion, pallor, and confusions connected with dialysis, can fundamentally influence a kid's day to day routine. Compelling side effect the executives, including the utilization of pharmacological intercessions, dietary help, and methodologies to alleviate the symptoms of medicines, adds to worked on actual prosperity. The objective is to limit the weight of side effects, permitting pediatric patients to lead more dynamic, agreeable, and side effect free lives notwithstanding the difficulties presented by renal problems.

3. **Psychosocial Effect and Psychological wellness:**
   The psychosocial effect of renal problems on pediatric patients is a basic part of personal satisfaction contemplations. Kids going through dialysis or living with CKD might encounter elevated degrees of stress, nervousness, and close to home misery. The interruption to typical youth exercises, expected sensations of confinement, and the familiarity with ongoing medical issue can affect emotional well-being. Psychosocial support, directing administrations, and the association of kid life experts are essential parts of tending to the psychosocial effect of renal problems. Personal satisfaction enhancements in this domain include encouraging a good psychological well-being climate, enabling youngsters to communicate their sentiments, and giving devices to adapt the personal difficulties related with renal circumstances.

4. **Instructive Coherence and Backing:**
   Guaranteeing instructive progression and backing is a critical thought in improving the personal satisfaction for pediatric patients with renal problems.
   The difficulties presented by dialysis plans, clinical arrangements, and potential hospitalizations might affect standard school participation. Personal satisfaction upgrades include teaming up with instructors, executing adaptable learning plans, and giving assets to locally situated schooling. The objective is to enable pediatric patients to proceed with their instructive interests, keep a feeling of predictability, and accomplish scholarly achievements notwithstanding the disturbances brought about by renal problems and their medicines.

5. **Relational peculiarities and Parental figure Prosperity:**
   Relational peculiarities assume a pivotal part in the personal satisfaction of pediatric patients confronting renal difficulties. The effect of renal problems reaches out past the impacted youngster to the whole family, affecting parental figure jobs, obligations, and prosperity. Personal satisfaction contemplations include supporting parental figures through instructive assets, relief care, and psychosocial mediations. Enabling families to explore the difficulties related with pediatric renal issues adds to a more strong climate, encouraging strength, and emphatically influencing the general personal satisfaction for both the kid and their guardians.

6. **Healthful Administration and Dietary Guiding:**
   Dietary contemplations are central in pediatric nephrology, and compelling administration assumes a crucial part in improving the personal satisfaction for youthful patients. Dietary limitations, liquid admission limits, and the requirement for particular healthful help are familiar parts of renal consideration. Personal satisfaction enhancements include customized dietary guiding, coordinated effort with dietitians, and the

combination of nourishing intercessions that line up with the youngster's age, inclinations, and generally wellbeing objectives. By tending to healthful requirements, pediatric patients can encounter further developed energy levels, better development results, and an improved feeling of prosperity.

7. **Change to Renal Transplantation:**
The quest for renal transplantation addresses a huge achievement in the personal satisfaction venture for pediatric patients with renal issues. Changing from dialysis to renal transplantation offers the commitment of reestablished kidney capability, decreased treatment troubles, and the potential for a more typical life. Personal satisfaction enhancements in this setting include extensive pre-relocate assessments, coordination among dialysis and relocate groups, and progressing support during the post-relocate period. Fruitful renal transplantation is a groundbreaking victory, denoting a shift towards worked on personal satisfaction, expanded independence, and the quest for long haul prosperity.

8. **All encompassing Ways to deal with Pediatric Nephrology Care:**
All encompassing ways to deal with pediatric nephrology care accentuate far reaching care that goes past the administration of actual side effects. Incorporating psychosocial support, instructive intercessions, and healthful administration into the general consideration plan adds to personal satisfaction improvements.

The comprehensive methodology perceives the interconnectedness of physical, close to home, and social prosperity, and tries to address the special requirements of every kid with regards to their family and local area. Personal satisfaction upgrades arise when pediatric nephrology care is custom-made to the singular necessities of the kid, remembering them as entire people as opposed to only patients with renal problems.

9. **Exploration and Advancement in Pediatric Nephrology:**
Personal satisfaction contemplations in pediatric nephrology are persistently developing with continuous exploration and advancement. Progressions in treatment modalities, dialysis innovation, and renal transplantation procedures add to further developed results and improved personal satisfaction for youthful patients. Research tries pointed toward figuring out the drawn out effect of renal issues, creating designated intercessions, and tending to the particular necessities of pediatric populaces impel the field forward. Personal satisfaction upgrades are unpredictably connected to the consistent development of pediatric nephrology rehearses through examination, advancement, and a pledge to improving results.

10. **Peer Backing and Local area Commitment:**
Building a feeling of local area and cultivating peer support contribute

essentially to the personal satisfaction for pediatric patients with renal problems. Interfacing youthful patients with others confronting comparative difficulties makes a steady organization where shared encounters, counsel, and consolation become important assets. Local area commitment drives, support gatherings, and valuable open doors for social collaboration add to improved psychosocial prosperity and a feeling of having a place. Personal satisfaction improvements in this domain perceive the significance of building a local area that comprehends and upholds the extraordinary excursion of pediatric patients in the domain of nephrology.

11. **Support for Pediatric Renal Wellbeing:**
Support endeavors assume a vital part in molding the scene of pediatric nephrology and improving the personal satisfaction for youthful patients. Backing drives plan to bring issues to light about renal problems, secure subsidizing for exploration, and impact medical services approaches that focus on pediatric renal wellbeing. By supporting for expanded admittance to mind, diminished incongruities, and the joining of personal satisfaction contemplations into medical services arrangements, advocates add to a climate where pediatric patients get thorough and comprehensive consideration.

12. **Kept Checking and Transformation:**

Personal satisfaction contemplations in pediatric nephrology require continuous observing and transformation. Customary evaluations of the physical, psychosocial, and instructive parts of a youngster's life add to a powerful consideration plan that advances as the kid develops and creates. The capacity to adjust mediations, address arising difficulties, and celebrate achievements addresses a continuous obligation to upgrading the general personal satisfaction for pediatric patients confronting renal issues.

CHAPTER 5

Genetic and Inherited Kidney Disorders

Hereditary and acquired kidney problems address a different gathering of conditions that can influence people from earliest stages through adulthood. These issues are portrayed by transformations or irregularities in unambiguous qualities, prompting underlying and utilitarian changes in the kidneys. Understanding the hereditary premise of kidney problems is fundamental for conclusion, visualization, and the improvement of designated remedial mediations. This investigation digs into the intricacies of hereditary and acquired kidney issues, analyzing the hidden systems, normal circumstances, demonstrative methodologies, and the developing scene of hereditary medication in nephrology.

1. **Hereditary Premise and Systems:**
   Hereditary kidney problems emerge from changes or modifications in the DNA arrangement of explicit qualities associated with kidney advancement, capability, or support. The hereditary premise can differ broadly, incorporating single quality changes, chromosomal anomalies, and complex hereditary communications.

   These changes might influence proteins engaged with renal filtration, cylindrical capability, electrolyte balance, or the underlying uprightness of the kidneys. Acquired kidney issues can be sorted in view of the method of legacy, including autosomal predominant, autosomal latent, X-connected, or mitochondrial designs. The different hereditary components add to the heterogeneity of clinical introductions and results seen in hereditary kidney issues.

2. **Normal Hereditary Kidney Problems:**
   A few hereditary kidney problems have been distinguished, each described by particular clinical highlights and fundamental hereditary transformations. One noticeable model is autosomal predominant polycystic kidney

sickness (ADPKD), a condition essentially brought about by changes in the PKD1 or PKD2 qualities. ADPKD prompts the development of liquid filled blisters in the kidneys, at last affecting renal capability. Autosomal passive polycystic kidney illness (ARPKD), another cystic kidney problem, regularly presents in earliest stages and results from transformations in the PKHD1 quality. Alport condition, described by glomerular irregularities and sensorineural hearing misfortune, is frequently connected to transformations in collagen qualities, like COL4A3, COL4A4, and COL4A5. These address only a couple of models, underscoring the hereditary variety inside the range of acquired kidney problems.

3. **Clinical Introductions and Phenotypic Changeability:**
The clinical introductions of hereditary kidney problems show huge phenotypic fluctuation, even among people with a similar fundamental hereditary transformation. This inconstancy is affected by elements like the particular transformation, natural impacts, and hereditary modifiers. At times, people with indistinguishable hereditary transformations might show various periods of beginning, paces of sickness movement, and seriousness of side effects. Phenotypic changeability presents difficulties in anticipating sickness results and highlights the requirement for customized ways to deal with analysis, the executives, and hereditary directing.

4. **Indicative Methodologies:**
The analysis of hereditary kidney problems has developed with progressions in hereditary testing advances. Sub-atomic hereditary testing, including methods, for example, DNA sequencing and designated quality boards, assumes a focal part in distinguishing pathogenic changes. Hereditary testing can affirm a clinical determination, work with forecast, guide treatment choices, and illuminate family arranging. At times, hereditary testing might be started in light of clinical doubt, while in others, it could be provoked by a family background of renal issues. Furthermore, high level imaging modalities, for example, renal ultrasound and attractive reverberation imaging (X-ray), supplement hereditary testing by giving bits of knowledge into the primary changes inside the kidneys.

5. **Hereditary Guiding and Family Arranging:**
Hereditary directing is a critical part of the consideration gave to people and families impacted by hereditary kidney problems.
Hereditary instructors work intimately with medical care groups to pass on complex hereditary data, examine legacy designs, and survey the gamble of passing the condition to people in the future. The coordination of hereditary directing into the indicative cycle enables people and families to arrive at informed conclusions about family arranging, pre-birth testing, and the expected ramifications of hereditary kidney problems for people in the future. As hereditary testing turns out to be more modern,

the job of hereditary advising turns out to be progressively significant in exploring the intricacies of acquired renal circumstances.

6. **Propels in Accuracy Medication:**
The period of accuracy medication has introduced extraordinary ways to deal with the finding and the board of hereditary kidney issues. Accuracy medication tailors remedial mediations in light of the one of a kind hereditary cosmetics of every person. With regards to hereditary nephrology, this might include the advancement of designated treatments pointed toward revising or relieving the impacts of explicit hereditary changes. The recognizable proof of hereditary modifiers, which impact the phenotypic articulation of hereditary issues, further upgrades the potential for accuracy medication intercessions. The developing scene of accuracy medication holds guarantee for further developed results, customized treatment plans, and novel remedial systems in the domain of hereditary kidney issues.

7. **Quality Treatments and Arising Intercessions:**
The investigation of quality treatments addresses a boondocks in the field of hereditary kidney issues. Quality treatment plans to address the underlying driver of hereditary changes by presenting utilitarian qualities or altering the outflow of defective qualities. While quality treatments are still in the beginning phases of improvement, promising headways have been made in preclinical examinations and clinical preliminaries. As the comprehension of the atomic systems basic hereditary kidney problems extends, quality treatments might offer designated mediations that adjust sickness movement, lighten side effects, or even give fixes from now on.

8. **Challenges in Hereditary Medication:**
Notwithstanding the promising advancements in hereditary medication, challenges continue in the successful interpretation of hereditary disclosures into clinical practice. The recognizable proof of hereditary changes doesn't generally relate with the seriousness or consistency of sickness results. Also, the intricacy of hereditary associations, natural elements, and the impact of hereditary modifiers present difficulties in precisely anticipating the clinical course of hereditary kidney issues. Moral contemplations, including issues connected with hereditary security, assent, and the potential psychosocial effect of hereditary data, additionally add to the difficulties related with the reconciliation of hereditary medication into routine nephrology care.

9. **Acquired Kidney Issues in Pediatric Nephrology:**
The effect of hereditary kidney problems is especially critical in the pediatric nephrology setting. Kids impacted by acquired renal circumstances might confront long lasting difficulties, including the possible requirement for renal substitution treatments, continuous clinical administration, and

the psychosocial ramifications of an ongoing hereditary condition. Early determination, far reaching the board plans, and family-focused care are fundamental parts of tending to the one of a kind requirements of pediatric patients with acquired kidney issues. Cooperative endeavors between pediatric nephrologists, geneticists, and hereditary guides add to a comprehensive way to deal with care for kids and their families.

10. **Research Wildernesses and Cooperative Drives:**
The investigation of hereditary and acquired kidney problems is a functioning area of exploration, described by cooperative drives and multidisciplinary approaches. Research attempts center around explaining the sub-atomic systems of hereditary changes, recognizing novel helpful targets, and understanding the elements adding to phenotypic inconstancy. Cooperative drives including worldwide consortia, research organizations, and patient support bunches add to the aggregate information base and speed up progressions in the field. The coordination of hereditary investigation into clinical practice holds the possibility to upset the conclusion, the executives, and treatment of hereditary kidney issues.

11. **Patient Strengthening and Backing:**
Patient strengthening and backing assume urgent parts in the scene of hereditary kidney issues. People and families impacted by these circumstances frequently become advocates for expanded mindfulness, research financing, and further developed admittance to hereditary testing and directing. Patient promotion bunches give a stage to sharing encounters, encouraging local area support, and impacting strategy changes. By effectively captivating in backing endeavors, people with hereditary kidney problems add to the more extensive exchange encompassing uncommon illnesses, hereditary exploration, and the significance of customized care.

12. **Future Headings and Comprehensive Consideration:**

The fate of hereditary nephrology holds invigorating conceivable outcomes, from the refinement of demonstrative apparatuses to the improvement of designated treatments and possible fixes. All encompassing consideration moves toward that coordinate hereditary data into complete consideration plans will be fundamental in tending to the assorted requirements of people with acquired kidney problems. The joining of hereditary medication into routine nephrology practice, combined with progressing research, cooperative endeavors, and patient-focused care, will shape the direction of hereditary nephrology in the years to come.

5.1 Understanding Genetic Factors in Pediatric Nephrology
Understanding hereditary variables in pediatric nephrology is fundamental for unwinding the intricacies of renal wellbeing in youngsters and youths.

Hereditary impacts assume a critical part in the turn of events, capability, and upkeep of the kidneys, adding to a range of renal problems that can show right off the bat throughout everyday life. This investigation dives into the unpredictable scene of hereditary variables in pediatric nephrology, enveloping the hereditary premise of renal turn of events, normal hereditary kidney issues in youngsters, progressions in hereditary diagnostics, the effect on clinical consideration, and the developing worldview of customized medication in the field.

1. **Hereditary Premise of Renal Turn of events:**
   The underpinning of renal wellbeing starts during undeveloped turn of events, where a progression of many-sided hereditary occasions coordinate the development and separation of the kidneys. Key flagging pathways, like those including WNT, BMP, and Score, manage the destiny of renal begetter cells and add to the advancement of nephrons, the practical units of the kidneys. Disturbances in these hereditary pathways can prompt inherent irregularities of the kidneys and urinary parcel (CAKUT), a different gathering of conditions that influence the design and capability of the kidneys. Understanding the hereditary variables engaged with renal advancement gives bits of knowledge into the beginnings of inborn kidney issues saw in pediatric nephrology.

2. **Normal Hereditary Kidney Issues in Youngsters:**
   Hereditary variables contribute altogether to different kidney issues that manifest in adolescence. Autosomal predominant polycystic kidney sickness (ADPKD), frequently brought about by changes in the PKD1 or PKD2 qualities, is one such model. ADPKD is portrayed by the development of liquid filled sores in the kidneys, prompting moderate renal brokenness. Autosomal passive polycystic kidney sickness (ARPKD), coming about because of transformations in the PKHD1 quality, regularly presents in early stages and is related with cystic changes in the kidneys. Alport condition, a hereditary problem influencing the glomerular cellar layer, is frequently brought about by changes in collagen qualities like COL4A3, COL4A4, and COL4A5. These models highlight the assorted hereditary scene of kidney problems influencing youngsters.

3. **Propels in Hereditary Diagnostics:**
   The coming of cutting edge hereditary diagnostics has upset the way to deal with distinguishing and figuring out hereditary elements in pediatric nephrology. Sub-atomic hereditary testing, including strategies, for example, DNA sequencing and designated quality boards, empowers the identification of pathogenic changes related with different kidney problems.
   Entire exome sequencing and entire genome sequencing offer extensive

examinations of the whole protein-coding locales or the whole genome, separately, giving a useful asset to revealing hereditary variations. The use of these innovations has worked with exact and early analyses, taking into account ideal intercessions and customized administration plans for youngsters with hereditary kidney issues.

4. **Influence on Clinical Consideration:**
The coordination of hereditary data into clinical consideration has extraordinary ramifications for pediatric nephrology. Hereditary determinations empower medical care suppliers to tailor the executives systems in light of the fundamental hereditary elements impacting a kid's renal wellbeing. This customized approach stretches out past treatment choices, affecting visualization, family arranging contemplations, and the expectation of likely intricacies. Hereditary data can direct the recurrence and force of observing, illuminate decisions connected with renal substitution treatments, and add to the general complete consideration of pediatric patients with hereditary kidney issues.

5. **Hereditary Elements in Inborn Abnormalities:**
Inherent irregularities of the kidneys and urinary lot (CAKUT) include a range of primary irregularities that emerge during fetal turn of events. Hereditary elements assume a vital part in the pathogenesis of CAKUT, impacting the development of renal designs and their network with the urinary lot. Changes in qualities engaged with renal advancement pathways, for example, RET, HNF1B, and PAX2, have been embroiled in CAKUT. The comprehension of hereditary variables adding to CAKUT improves the capacity to foresee and deal with these abnormalities, working with early mediations to save renal capability in impacted youngsters.

6. **Effect of Hereditary Elements on Infection Movement:**
Hereditary variables not just add to the underlying improvement of kidney problems yet additionally impact the direction of sickness movement. Fluctuation in the seriousness and pace of movement of hereditary kidney problems is frequently owing to the particular hereditary changes included. Also, the ID of hereditary modifiers, which can improve or constrict the impacts of essential hereditary transformations, further adds to the intricacy of infection results. Unwinding the complexities of hereditary elements impacting sickness movement improves prognostic capacities, empowering medical services suppliers to successfully expect and oversee inconveniences.

7. **Exploring Hereditary Intricacy in Pediatric Patients:**
Pediatric nephrologists face the test of exploring the hereditary intricacy innate in pediatric patients with kidney issues. The phenotypic fluctuation saw among people with indistinguishable hereditary transformations requires a nuanced way to deal with patient consideration.

Factors like hereditary modifiers, natural impacts, and individual hereditary foundations add to this intricacy. Cooperative endeavors between pediatric nephrologists, geneticists, and hereditary instructors are fundamental for unraveling this intricacy, guaranteeing exact analyses, and figuring out custom-made administration designs that address the novel necessities of every kid.

8. **Suggestions for Family Arranging:**
Understanding hereditary elements in pediatric nephrology has significant ramifications for family arranging. Families with a background marked by hereditary kidney problems might look for hereditary directing to evaluate the gamble of giving the condition to people in the future. Hereditary guides assume a crucial part in passing on complex hereditary data, examining legacy designs, and helping families in pursuing informed choices. The mix of hereditary data into family arranging contemplations enables people and families to pursue decisions lined up with their qualities and inclinations, cultivating informed direction and lessening the gamble of genetic kidney problems in ensuing ages.

9. **Unwinding the Atomic Premise of Hereditary Issues:**
Progressions in sub-atomic hereditary qualities have worked with the unwinding of the atomic premise of different hereditary kidney problems. The ID of explicit hereditary changes liable for conditions like ADPKD, ARPKD, and Alport disorder has extended how we might interpret the fundamental pathophysiology. This sub-atomic understanding gives an establishment to the improvement of designated treatments pointed toward tending to the underlying driver of these problems. By explaining the sub-atomic pathways included, specialists and clinicians can investigate imaginative intercessions that might change sickness movement and further develop results for impacted youngsters.

10. **Customized Medication in Pediatric Nephrology:**
The worldview of customized medication is progressively acquiring conspicuousness in pediatric nephrology, driven by propels in hereditary diagnostics and sub-atomic comprehension. Customized medication tailors treatment plans to the novel hereditary cosmetics of every person, enhancing remedial mediations in light of their hereditary profile. This approach holds extraordinary commitment for hereditary kidney issues, offering the potential for designated treatments that address the particular components adding to infection pathogenesis. As examination in this field advances, the execution of customized medication approaches can possibly upset the consideration of pediatric patients with hereditary kidney problems.

11. **Research Outskirts in Pediatric Nephrology:**
Progressing research tries in pediatric nephrology center around extend-

ing our insight into hereditary elements impacting renal wellbeing in youngsters. Cooperative exploration organizations, global consortia, and multidisciplinary studies add to the aggregate comprehension of the hereditary scene of pediatric kidney problems.

Propels in advancements, for example, CRISPR quality altering and single-cell genomics hold guarantee for additional clarifying the sub-atomic complexities of hereditary kidney issues and investigating imaginative helpful roads. The crossing point of hereditary qualities, atomic science, and clinical exploration keeps on molding the outskirts of information in pediatric nephrology.

12. **Moral Contemplations and Hereditary Protection:**

As hereditary data becomes basic to pediatric nephrology care, moral contemplations encompassing hereditary protection and agree come to the front. Defending the classification of hereditary data, acquiring informed assent for hereditary testing, and exploring the psychosocial effect of hereditary judgments are fundamental parts of moral practice. Pediatric nephrologists, hereditary advocates, and medical services groups should focus on moral contemplations in coordinating hereditary data into clinical consideration, guaranteeing that families are upheld, enabled, and completely educated all through the analytic and helpful excursion.

5.2 Challenges in Genetic Counseling

Hereditary directing assumes a urgent part in the field of hereditary qualities and medical services, giving people and families data about the legacy of hereditary issues, the related dangers, and the accessible choices for overseeing and forestalling these circumstances. While hereditary directing is a significant and fundamental help, it isn't without its difficulties. This investigation digs into the multi-layered difficulties looked by hereditary advisors, enveloping the intricacy of hereditary data, moral contemplations, the effect on people and families, social responsiveness, the advancing scene of hereditary testing, and the requirement for continuous expert training and backing.

1. **Intricacy of Hereditary Data:**
   Hereditary data is intrinsically perplexing, including unpredictable atomic cycles, legacy examples, and potential wellbeing suggestions. Imparting this intricacy to people who might not have experience with hereditary qualities represents a huge test for hereditary guides. Adjusting the requirement for precision with the capacity to pass on data in an unmistakable and reasonable way requires expertise and responsiveness. Hereditary instructors should distil complex hereditary ideas into edible data, guaranteeing that people and families can settle on informed

conclusions about their medical services in light of an exhaustive comprehension of their hereditary dangers.

2. **Profound Effect on People and Families:**
Hereditary directing frequently manages data that can have significant close to home ramifications for people and families. Finding out about a hereditary inclination to a condition or the gamble of giving a hereditary issue to people in the future can sincerely challenge.

Hereditary instructors should explore the close to home scene with compassion, offering help and direction while regarding the extraordinary survival strategies of every person. Adjusting the conveyance of possibly upsetting data with the requirement for everyday encouragement is a fragile part of the hereditary guiding cycle.

3. **Moral Contemplations and Informed Assent:**
Hereditary directing is innately attached to moral contemplations, especially in regards to informed assent. Giving people extensive data about hereditary testing, possible results, and the ramifications for them as well as their families is fundamental for guaranteeing independence and informed direction. In any case, accomplishing educated assent in the setting regarding complex hereditary data requires cautious consideration regarding the singular's comprehension, guaranteeing that they understand the idea of the hereditary testing, the expected outcomes, and the ramifications for their medical services choices.

4. **Psychosocial and Social Responsiveness:**
Social and psychosocial factors fundamentally impact how people see and answer hereditary data. Hereditary guides should be sensitive to the different social foundations, conviction frameworks, and social settings of the people they serve. Social awareness includes recognizing and regarding social contrasts, fitting correspondence to line up with social standards, and tending to the psychosocial effect of hereditary data inside social systems. Aversion to social variety guarantees that hereditary advising administrations are open, deferential, and receptive to the interesting necessities of different populaces.

5. **Effect of Vulnerability:**
Hereditary testing doesn't necessarily in every case give conclusive responses, and vulnerability is inborn in some hereditary advising situations. Fluctuation in the penetrance of specific hereditary variations, questionable outcomes, or the absence of distinguished causative transformations can make difficulties in passing on clear and certain data. Hereditary guides should actually convey the degree of vulnerability while supporting people in going with choices in light of the accessible data. Overseeing vulnerability is a powerful part of hereditary directing

that requires continuous schooling and variation to arising hereditary information.

6. **Challenges in Pediatric Hereditary Advising:**
Pediatric hereditary directing presents extra intricacies, as the data influences the youngster as well as has ramifications for guardians and more distant family individuals. Tending to the feelings of guardians, passing on data in a kid cordial way, and including families in dynamic cycles are basic parts of pediatric hereditary directing. Hereditary advisors should explore the harmony between giving age-fitting data to the kid while guaranteeing that guardians have the information and backing expected to go with educated choices for benefit regarding their youngsters.

7. **Openness and Value:**
Guaranteeing fair admittance to hereditary directing administrations is a huge test in the field. Financial variables, geographic area, and variations in medical care access can make obstructions to getting hereditary guiding administrations. The test isn't just in offering types of assistance yet in addition in fitting them to assorted populaces, considering etymological, social, and proficiency factors. Endeavors to upgrade availability and value in hereditary guiding include local area effort, schooling, and the advancement of socially equipped assets that address the requirements of various populaces.

8. **Staying up with Mechanical Advances:**
The field of hereditary qualities is quickly developing, with continuous innovative advances adding to the disclosure of new hereditary markers, indicative apparatuses, and treatment choices. Hereditary instructors face the test of keeping up to date with these progressions, figuring out their clinical ramifications, and integrating them into their training. Staying up with innovation includes consistent training, proficient turn of events, and cooperation with geneticists, scientists, and other medical services experts to guarantee that hereditary advising stays educated and viable.

9. **Protection and Hereditary Information Security:**
The idea of hereditary data raises worries about protection and information security. Hereditary advocates handle delicate and individual data that, whenever misused, could have critical ramifications for people and families. Guaranteeing powerful information safety efforts, complying to security guidelines, and imparting obviously about the privacy of hereditary data are fundamental parts of moral hereditary directing practice. Keeping up with the trust and certainty of people in the security of their hereditary information is pivotal for the fruitful conveyance of hereditary directing administrations.

10. **Consolidating Genomic Schooling in Clinical Preparation:**
The mix of hereditary qualities into standard medical care requires a

purposeful work to consolidate genomic schooling into the preparation of medical services experts, including hereditary guides. Challenges emerge in guaranteeing that clinical experts across different claims to fame have a central comprehension of hereditary qualities and can successfully team up with hereditary guides. Support for the consideration of genomic schooling in clinical educational plans, continuous preparation drives, and interdisciplinary cooperation are fundamental parts of tending to this test.

11. **Tending to Disgrace and Misguided judgments:**
Hereditary circumstances, particularly those with noticeable indications, might be related with disgrace and confusions. Hereditary guides assume a pivotal part in tending to and dissipating disgrace, advancing precise data, and cultivating understanding inside networks.
Teaching people and families about the idea of hereditary problems, underlining the variety of hereditary circumstances, and testing misguided judgments add to establishing a more educated and steady climate.

12. **Proficient Prosperity and Burnout:**

The profound force of hereditary guiding, combined with the obligation of passing on possibly life changing data, can add to proficient burnout. Hereditary guides should explore the profound cost of their work, take part in taking care of oneself practices, and approach steady conditions. Laying out instruments for peer backing, oversight, and continuous expert advancement is urgent for supporting the prosperity of hereditary advisors and guaranteeing the proceeded with conveyance of top notch care.

5.3 Triumphs in Genetic Therapies and Interventions

Wins in hereditary treatments and mediations address a groundbreaking time in medication, offering extraordinary chances to address the main drivers of hereditary problems and change treatment draws near. As logical comprehension of hereditary qualities develops, imaginative treatments are arising to address or relieve the impacts of hereditary transformations, achieving wins in the domain of accuracy medication. This investigation dives into the wonderful advancement and wins in hereditary treatments, enveloping quality altering innovations, quality treatments, triumphs in clinical preliminaries, moral contemplations, and the possible effect on a range of hereditary problems.

1. **Quality Altering Innovations:**
Quality altering innovations have arisen as incredible assets for unequivocally adjusting the DNA groupings inside the genome, offering the possibility to address hereditary transformations at the sub-atomic level. CRISPR-Cas9, specifically, has altered quality altering, taking into

consideration designated adjustments with exceptional accuracy. Wins in quality altering advances incorporate the capacity to address pathogenic changes, embed helpful qualities, or tweak quality articulation to reestablish typical cell capability. The flexibility of these innovations holds guarantee for many hereditary problems, from monogenic circumstances to complex polygenic infections.

2. **Quality Treatments for Monogenic Problems:**
   One of the striking victories in hereditary mediations is the improvement of quality treatments for monogenic problems. Monogenic problems result from transformations in a solitary quality, prompting explicit practical deficiencies. Quality treatments intend to address these shortfalls by presenting practical duplicates of the impacted quality or regulating the declaration of related qualities. Remarkable triumphs incorporate medicines for acquired retinal issues, where quality treatments have shown the capacity to reestablish vision by revising hereditary changes influencing photoreceptor cells. These victories highlight the potential for quality treatments to give groundbreaking results to people impacted by a range of monogenic problems.

3. **Triumphs in Clinical Preliminaries:**
   Wins in hereditary treatments are obvious in fruitful results from clinical preliminaries, where creative mediations are thoroughly tried for well-being and viability. Clinical preliminaries have shown the attainability and adequacy of quality treatments in different hereditary issues, including hemophilia, solid dystrophy, and specific sorts of disease. Prominent victories incorporate the endorsement of Luxturna, a quality treatment for an uncommon type of acquired visual impairment, and Zolgensma, a quality treatment for spinal solid decay, stamping critical achievements in the interpretation of hereditary treatments from the research center to clinical practice.

4. **Forward leaps in Hematopoietic Undeveloped cell Treatments:**
   Hematopoietic undeveloped cell (HSC) treatments address a victory in the field of hereditary mediations, especially for messes influencing the blood and safe frameworks. In conditions like extreme joined immunodeficiency (SCID), ordinarily known as "bubble kid" illness, hematopoietic immature microorganism transplantation has been effective in giving a corrective methodology by supplanting deficient safe cells with solid ones. Progresses in quality altering advancements have additionally upgraded the capability of HSC treatments, considering exact rectification of hereditary changes in undifferentiated organisms before transplantation, limiting the gamble of entanglements and unite versus-have illness.

5. **Headways in Antisense Oligonucleotide Treatments:**
   Antisense oligonucleotide (ASO) treatments address a victory in the

domain of RNA-based mediations. ASOs are short manufactured nucleotides intended to specifically tie to target RNA groupings, balancing quality articulation and protein creation. This approach has shown outcome in treating specific hereditary issues, including Duchenne solid dystrophy and spinal strong decay. By adjusting the grafting of RNA or advancing exon skipping, ASO treatments mean to reestablish the development of useful proteins, alleviating the effect of pathogenic changes.

6. **Customized Malignant growth Therapapies:**
Hereditary mediations have yielded wins in the domain of customized disease treatments. The distinguishing proof of explicit hereditary changes driving disease development has made ready for designated treatments custom-made to the hereditary profile of individual growths. Tyrosine kinase inhibitors, immunotherapies, and other accuracy medication approaches have shown astounding outcome in treating different kinds of disease. The capacity to target explicit hereditary modifications in malignant growth cells while saving ordinary cells addresses a victory in limiting secondary effects and further developing treatment results.

7. **Moral Contemplations in Hereditary Treatments:**
The victories in hereditary treatments likewise deliver moral contemplations that require cautious route. The moral ramifications of quality altering, especially germline altering that influences people in the future, bring up issues about the possible potentially negative side-effects and the requirement for dependable utilization of these advances. Finding some kind of harmony between logical advancement and moral protections includes progressing discourse, worldwide coordinated effort, and the improvement of moral rules to guarantee that hereditary treatments are applied in a way that focuses on security, value, and regard for human nobility.

8. **Access and Reasonableness:**
While wins in hereditary treatments offer extraordinary potential, guaranteeing far and wide access and reasonableness stays a test. The turn of events and creation of quality treatments can be asset concentrated, prompting significant expenses that might restrict availability for specific populaces. Resolving issues of access and reasonableness includes exploring medical services frameworks, drawing in with drug organizations, and investigating creative methodologies, for example, repayment models in light of long haul results. The moral basic to make these groundbreaking treatments open to an expansive populace stays a basic thought.

9. **Tending to Difficulties in Quality Conveyance:**
Wins in hereditary treatments frequently depend on the fruitful conveyance of remedial qualities or quality altering devices to target cells. Challenges in quality conveyance incorporate issues connected with

the effectiveness of conveyance strategies, the potential for off-target impacts, and the resistant reaction set off by the presentation of unfamiliar hereditary material. Propels in viral vectors, nanoparticles, and other conveyance frameworks plan to improve the accuracy and security of quality conveyance, defeating obstructions that might restrict the adequacy of hereditary treatments.

10. **Long haul Toughness of Hereditary Intercessions:**
Surveying the drawn out solidness of hereditary mediations addresses a continuous test in the field. While a few hereditary treatments have shown progress in giving supported benefits, questions stay about the constancy of remedial impacts over a singular's life expectancy. Checking the drawn out results of people who go through hereditary mediations is fundamental for figuring out the sturdiness of these treatments and refining ways to deal with guarantee enduring advantages.

11. **Defeating Safe Reactions:**
The safe framework's reaction to hereditary treatments presents difficulties that should be tended to for supported achievement.
Resistant responses to viral vectors or restorative proteins can affect the viability of quality treatments and may present wellbeing concerns. Creating systems to balance safe reactions, upgrade the decency of helpful mediations, and limit the gamble of unfavorable responses addresses a continuous area of examination and refinement in the field of hereditary treatments.

12. **Continuous Expert Schooling and Cooperation:**

The quick speed of headways in hereditary treatments requires continuous expert training and joint effort among medical care suppliers, scientists, and hereditary advisors. Staying informed concerning developing innovations, grasping the most recent clinical preliminary results, and remaining informed about moral contemplations require a pledge to nonstop learning. Interdisciplinary cooperation is fundamental for encouraging an aggregate comprehension of hereditary treatments and their suggestions for different clinical strengths, guaranteeing that medical care experts are prepared to incorporate these victories into routine clinical practice.

CHAPTER 6

Pediatric Hypertension

Pediatric hypertension, a condition described by raised circulatory strain in youngsters and youths, has arisen as a huge wellbeing worry with suggestions for long haul cardiovascular wellbeing. While hypertension is frequently connected with grown-ups, its presence in the pediatric populace requires cautious consideration and the executives. This investigation dives into the complex scene of pediatric hypertension, including its pervasiveness, risk factors, demonstrative difficulties, fundamental causes, possible entanglements, and the significance of early intercession for ideal long haul wellbeing results.

1. **Commonness of Pediatric Hypertension:**
   Pediatric hypertension is progressively perceived as a common medical problem. The commonness rates shift across various populaces and are affected by elements like age, orientation, and identity. As per the American Foundation of Pediatrics (AAP), it is assessed that roughly 3.5% of all kids and young people in the US have hypertension. The predominance is higher among specific subgroups, incorporating those with heftiness or a family background of hypertension. The increasing paces of experience growing up corpulence, inactive ways of life, and dietary elements add to the expanded pervasiveness of pediatric hypertension, raising worries about its effect on general wellbeing.

2. **Risk Factors and Contributing Elements:**
   A few gamble factors add to the improvement of pediatric hypertension, with corpulence being a conspicuous and modifiable variable. Youngsters and teenagers with abundance body weight are at an expanded gamble of hypertension because of the transaction of metabolic elements, insulin opposition, and changes in the renin-angiotensin-aldosterone framework. Other gamble factors incorporate a family background of hypertension, low birth weight, untimely birth, and certain ailments like persistent

kidney sickness or diabetes. Dietary variables, especially unreasonable sodium consumption, and stationary ways of behaving further compound the gamble, accentuating the significance of extensive way of life alterations in hypertension anticipation and the board.

3. **Challenges in Conclusion:**
Diagnosing hypertension in youngsters presents remarkable difficulties contrasted with grown-ups. Pulse values shift with age, level, and orientation, requiring the utilization old enough unambiguous percentiles to characterize hypertension in youngsters. The determination is affirmed when pulse estimations reliably surpass the 95th percentile for age, orientation, and level on numerous events. Wandering circulatory strain observing and home pulse estimations are significant devices in beating the difficulties of white coat hypertension and giving a more precise evaluation of a kid's circulatory strain profile. Be that as it may, the absence of routine pulse checking in well-kid visits and the fluctuation in estimation procedures add to the underdiagnosis and undertreatment of pediatric hypertension.

4. **Fundamental Causes and Auxiliary Hypertension:**
While essential or fundamental hypertension, frequently connected to way of life factors, is normal in kids, optional hypertension emerging from a hidden ailment is a basic thought. Optional hypertension represents a critical extent of cases in the pediatric populace and requires exhaustive assessment to recognize and address the main driver. Renal parenchymal illness, coarctation of the aorta, endocrine issues (like hyperthyroidism or hyperaldosteronism), and certain drugs are among the bunch reasons for optional hypertension. The recognizable proof of optional hypertension is significant for directing designated mediations and forestalling long haul inconveniences.

5. **Likely Difficulties and Cardiovascular Dangers:**
Untreated or ineffectively controlled pediatric hypertension can prompt different complexities and stances long haul cardiovascular dangers. Determined height of pulse overburdens the vascular framework, adding to the early improvement of atherosclerosis and cardiovascular rebuilding. The effect of hypertension on track organs, including the heart, kidneys, and veins, may bring about end-organ harm. Moreover, hypertensive kids are at an expanded gamble of growing left ventricular hypertrophy, a condition related with unfriendly cardiovascular results in adulthood. Early mediation is principal to moderate these dangers and shield the cardiovascular soundness of impacted people all through their life expectancy.

6. **Way of life Adjustments and Non-Pharmacological Mediations:**
Way of life adjustments structure the foundation of pediatric hypertension the executives, especially in instances of essential hypertension.

Mediations center around advancing sound dietary propensities, expanding actual work, and accomplishing and keeping a solid weight. Dietary sodium limitation is stressed, as overabundance sodium admission adds to expanded circulatory strain. Conduct mediations, including family-based approaches, are instrumental in cultivating manageable way of life changes. Connecting with kids and their families in schooling and backing programs upgrades adherence to way of life changes, tending to the main drivers of pediatric hypertension.

7. **Pharmacological Mediations:**
In situations where way of life alterations alone are deficient, pharmacological mediations might be important to accomplish pulse control. The choice of antihypertensive drugs is directed by the basic reason for hypertension, comorbidities, and individual patient qualities. Regularly involved antihypertensive specialists in pediatric populaces incorporate angiotensin-changing over catalyst (Pro) inhibitors, angiotensin II receptor blockers (ARBs), calcium channel blockers, and diuretics. The inception and titration of drugs require close observing and joint effort between medical care suppliers, youngsters, and their families to guarantee ideal adequacy and limit possible secondary effects.

8. **Significance of Early Mediation:**
Early mediation in pediatric hypertension is of foremost significance to forestall the movement of the condition and alleviate long haul cardiovascular dangers. The ID and the executives of hypertension during youth establish the groundwork for a better adulthood. Routine pulse checking in well-kid visits, expanded mindfulness among medical care suppliers, and local area level drives pointed toward elevating sound ways of life add to early location and mediation. Family commitment and schooling assume vital parts in executing way of life changes and sticking to treatment plans, cultivating a cooperative way to deal with pediatric hypertension the board.

9. **Long haul Checking and Change to Grown-up Care:**
Pediatric hypertension requires long haul observing to evaluate treatment viability, address advancing gamble factors, and guarantee congruity of care into adulthood. The change from pediatric to grown-up care addresses a basic stage, requiring facilitated endeavors among pediatricians and grown-up medical services suppliers. Laying out a consistent progress plan guarantees that people with a background marked by pediatric hypertension get proper observing, continuous help, and mediations customized to their developing cardiovascular wellbeing needs. Joint effort among pediatric and grown-up medical services frameworks works with the trading of relevant clinical data and elevates a far reaching way to deal with long haul care.

10. **General Wellbeing Systems and Promotion:**
    Tending to pediatric hypertension requires a multi-layered general wellbeing approach enveloping support, training, and local area commitment. General wellbeing methodologies center around bringing issues to light among guardians, parental figures, and medical care suppliers about the significance of pulse observing in kids. School-based drives, local area wellbeing projects, and strategy intercessions pointed toward elevating sound conditions add to essential anticipation endeavors. Support for routine pulse separating kids, expanded admittance to medical care assets, and the execution of proof based mediations are fundamental parts of general wellbeing drives focusing on pediatric hypertension.

11. **Exploration and Advancement:**
    Progressions in examination and development assume a critical part in growing comprehension we might interpret pediatric hypertension and refining treatment draws near. Progressing research endeavors investigate the hereditary, ecological, and way of life factors affecting pulse guideline in youngsters. Developments in innovation, like wearable gadgets and telehealth stages, offer open doors for remote checking and upgraded correspondence between medical services suppliers and families. Cooperative exploration tries add to the advancement of proof based rules, illuminating accepted procedures for the finding and the board of pediatric hypertension.

12. **Tending to Abberations and Social Determinants:**

Pediatric hypertension meets with more extensive issues of wellbeing variations and social determinants of wellbeing. Financial elements, admittance to medical care assets, and natural impacts add to differences in the pervasiveness and the board of pediatric hypertension. Tending to these differences requires an exhaustive methodology that considers the social determinants impacting wellbeing results. Local area based intercessions, medical services strategy promotion, and designated drives pointed toward lessening wellbeing imbalances add to a more comprehensive and evenhanded way to deal with pediatric hypertension care.

6.1 Identifying and Managing Hypertension in Children

Distinguishing and overseeing hypertension in kids is a basic part of pediatric medical services, taking into account the possible long haul suggestions on cardiovascular wellbeing. While hypertension is usually connected with grown-ups, its presence in the pediatric populace requests cautious consideration, early location, and powerful mediation. This investigation digs into the intricacies of recognizing and overseeing hypertension in kids, enveloping the difficulties in conclusion, the significance of exact pulse estimations, hidden causes, way of life adjustments, pharmacological mediations, and the cooperative job of medical services suppliers, families, and the local area.

1. **Challenges in Finding:**
   Diagnosing hypertension in kids presents one of a kind difficulties contrasted with grown-ups. In contrast to grown-ups, where circulatory strain values are normalized and all around relevant, pediatric pulse fluctuates with age, level, and orientation. To address this inconstancy, pediatricians use age-explicit percentiles in view of standardizing information to characterize hypertension. The determination is affirmed when circulatory strain estimations reliably surpass the 95th percentile for age, orientation, and level on various events. Be that as it may, provokes emerge because of the absence of routine pulse observing in well-youngster visits, varieties in estimation strategies, and the peculiarity of white coat hypertension, where a kid's circulatory strain might ascend in a clinical setting because of nervousness.

2. **Significance of Precise Pulse Estimations:**
   Precise pulse estimations are basic to the ID and the board of hypertension in youngsters. Medical care suppliers should stick to normalized methods for pulse estimation, guaranteeing the utilization of appropriately measured sleeves, proper situating of the kid, and fastidious recording of readings. Perceiving the effect of natural elements, stress, and the potential for white coat hypertension, endeavors to make a quiet and happy with setting during pulse evaluations are vital. Furthermore, wandering pulse observing and home circulatory strain estimations give important bits of knowledge, conquering the impediments of single-point estimations and upgrading the precision of diagnosing pediatric hypertension.

3. **Hidden Reasons for Pediatric Hypertension:**
   Distinguishing the basic reasons for pediatric hypertension is fundamental for directing designated mediations. While essential or fundamental hypertension, frequently connected with way of life factors, is normal, a critical extent of cases include optional hypertension coming about because of a basic ailment. Renal parenchymal illness, coarctation of the aorta, endocrine problems (like hyperthyroidism or hyperaldosteronism), and certain drugs are among the heap reasons for auxiliary hypertension. An exhaustive assessment, including a careful clinical history, actual assessment, and research center tests, helps with pinpointing the underlying driver and deciding the most fitting strategy.

4. **Way of life Changes as a Foundation of The board:**
   Way of life adjustments structure the foundation of overseeing pediatric hypertension, especially in instances of essential hypertension. Intercessions center around advancing solid dietary propensities, expanding

actual work, and accomplishing and keeping a sound weight. Dietary sodium limitation is accentuated, as overabundance sodium consumption adds to raised circulatory strain. Conduct mediations, frequently including the family, assume a crucial part in cultivating feasible way of life changes. Cooperative endeavors between medical services suppliers and families to execute dietary adjustments, energize normal actual work, and address stationary ways of behaving add to successful administration and anticipation of pediatric hypertension.

5. **Pharmacological Intercessions When Essential:**
   In situations where way of life adjustments alone are lacking to accomplish pulse control, pharmacological mediations might be important. The determination of antihypertensive prescriptions is directed by the hidden reason for hypertension, the presence of comorbidities, and individual patient attributes. Usually involved antihypertensive specialists in pediatric populaces incorporate angiotensin-changing over catalyst (Pro) inhibitors, angiotensin II receptor blockers (ARBs), calcium channel blockers, and diuretics. The inception and titration of drugs require close observing and cooperation between medical services suppliers, kids, and their families to guarantee ideal adequacy and limit likely incidental effects.

6. **Cooperative Job of Medical care Suppliers:**
   Overseeing pediatric hypertension requires a cooperative methodology including medical services suppliers, kids, and their families. Pediatricians assume a focal part in routine circulatory strain checking during great kid visits, early recognizable proof of hypertension, and direction on way of life changes. Specific consideration from pediatric nephrologists, cardiologists, or endocrinologists might be looked for in instances of optional hypertension or complex ailments. Cooperative endeavors reach out to teaching families about the significance of adherence to treatment plans, way of life changes, and the drawn out ramifications of pediatric hypertension on cardiovascular wellbeing.

7. **Family Commitment and Instruction:**
   Connecting with families in the administration of pediatric hypertension is central for fruitful results. Training assumes a vital part in enabling guardians and parental figures to effectively take part in their kid's medical services venture. Families need to comprehend the meaning of routine pulse observing, the execution of way of life adjustments, and the reasoning behind pharmacological mediations when recommended. Open correspondence between medical care suppliers and families encourages a strong climate, guaranteeing that guardians are furnished with the information and assets expected to explore the intricacies of overseeing pediatric hypertension at home.

8. **Local area Contribution and General Wellbeing Drives:**
   Addressing pediatric hypertension reaches out past individual medical care settings to local area inclusion and general wellbeing drives. School-based programs, local area wellbeing efforts, and strategy intercessions add to essential avoidance endeavors. General wellbeing systems center around bringing issues to light among guardians, parental figures, and teachers about the significance of sound ways of life and routine circulatory strain checking in youngsters. Cooperative endeavors including schools, neighborhood wellbeing offices, and local area associations add to establishing conditions that advance actual work, smart dieting, and generally speaking cardiovascular prosperity.

9. **Exploration and Advances in Pediatric Hypertension:**
   Continuous examination assumes a urgent part in propelling comprehension we might interpret pediatric hypertension and refining treatment draws near. Research attempts investigate hereditary, natural, and way of life factors affecting circulatory strain guideline in kids. Advancements in innovation, like wearable gadgets and telehealth stages, offer open doors for remote checking and improved correspondence between medical care suppliers and families. Cooperative examination endeavors add to the improvement of proof based rules, illuminating accepted procedures for the analysis and the executives of pediatric hypertension.

10. **Occasional Checking and Progress to Grown-up Care:**
    Pediatric hypertension requires occasional checking to evaluate treatment viability, address developing gamble factors, and guarantee congruity of care into adulthood. The change from pediatric to grown-up care addresses a basic stage, requiring composed endeavors among pediatricians and grown-up medical services suppliers. Laying out a consistent progress plan guarantees that people with a background marked by pediatric hypertension get proper checking, continuous help, and mediations custom-made to their developing cardiovascular wellbeing needs. Joint effort among pediatric and grown-up medical services frameworks works with the trading of relevant clinical data and elevates an extensive way to deal with long haul care.

11. **Tending to Abberations and Social Determinants:**
    Pediatric hypertension meets with more extensive issues of wellbeing differences and social determinants of wellbeing. Financial elements, admittance to medical care assets, and natural impacts add to variations in the pervasiveness and the board of pediatric hypertension. Tending to these inconsistencies requires a thorough methodology that considers the social determinants impacting wellbeing results. Local area based intercessions, medical services strategy support, and designated drives pointed

toward diminishing wellbeing disparities add to a more comprehensive and impartial way to deal with pediatric hypertension care.

12. **Significance of Routine Well-Kid Visits:**

Routine well-kid visits act as a basic stage for the ID and the board of pediatric hypertension. Ordinary checking of pulse during great kid visits permits medical care suppliers to follow patterns, recognize potential issues early, and execute opportune intercessions. Well-kid visits additionally give open doors to schooling, guiding on way of life changes, and tending to any worries or questions raised by guardians or parental figures. Underlining the significance of routine well-youngster visits as an extensive procedure for pediatric medical services adds to the early recognition and powerful administration of hypertension in kids.

6.2 Challenges in Monitoring Blood Pressure in Pediatric Patients

Checking pulse in pediatric patients presents particular difficulties that require cautious thought and concentrated approaches. Dissimilar to grown-ups, kids' circulatory strain values are impacted by different variables, including age, level, and orientation. This intricacy, combined with the unique idea of pediatric physiology, requests a nuanced and extensive comprehension of the difficulties related with pulse observing in youngsters. This investigation digs into the extraordinary difficulties looked in checking pulse in pediatric patients, enveloping issues connected with regularizing information, the effect of development and improvement, the peculiarity of white coat hypertension, mechanical contemplations, and the significance of exact estimations for early location and compelling administration.

1. **Regulating Information and Age-Explicit Percentiles:**
   One of the essential difficulties in checking pulse in pediatric patients lies in the dependence on standardizing information and age-explicit percentiles. In contrast to grown-ups, where circulatory strain values are normalized, pediatric pulse differs with age, level, and orientation. Medical services suppliers use age-explicit percentiles got from regularizing information to characterize ordinary and unusual circulatory strain values in youngsters. This approach perceives the unique changes in circulatory strain over the course of growing up and youthfulness. Be that as it may, it likewise requires continuous reference to refreshed development diagrams and percentile tables to guarantee exact understanding, as standardizing values change with age and level.

2. **Effect of Development and Improvement:**
   The unique idea of development and improvement presents critical difficulties in circulatory strain observing for pediatric patients. Circulatory

strain values are affected by elements, for example, expanded weight, changes in heart result, and adjustments in vascular opposition as youngsters progress through various formative stages. Observing circulatory strain with regards to development requires a longitudinal methodology, taking into account the youngster's singular direction and representing varieties in pulse values related with ordinary development. Medical services suppliers should be proficient at deciphering pulse patterns after some time to recognize ordinary varieties and possible hypertension.

3. **White Coat Hypertension in Pediatric Patients:**
The peculiarity of white coat hypertension, where pulse readings are raised in a clinical setting because of uneasiness or stress, is especially important in pediatric patients. Youngsters might encounter elevated degrees of nervousness during clinical visits, prompting transient expansions in pulse.

Recognizing white coat hypertension and supported hypertension is fundamental for exact conclusion and suitable administration. Mobile pulse checking, which includes recording circulatory strain at customary stretches over the course of the constantly, gives a more exhaustive and exact evaluation, relieving the effect of white coat hypertension in pediatric patients.

4. **Absence of Routine Pulse Observing in Well-Kid Visits:**
In contrast to grown-ups, where routine pulse observing is a standard part of medical care visits, there is an absence of predictable and efficient circulatory strain checking in well-youngster visits for pediatric patients. This hole can add to underdiagnosis and undertreatment of hypertension in kids. Laying out routine circulatory strain estimations in well-kid visits is significant for early location, observing patterns, and executing opportune mediations. Coordinating circulatory strain observing into routine pediatric consideration makes a thorough way to deal with pediatric medical services, advancing cardiovascular wellbeing since the beginning.

5. **Age-Related Difficulties in Pulse Estimation:**
Pulse estimation procedures should be adjusted to the age and formative phase of the pediatric patient. Babies, little children, young kids, and youths might require various ways to deal with guarantee exact readings. The decision of sleeve size, situating of the youngster, and the determination of a fitting circulatory strain gadget all add to the precision of estimations. Medical services suppliers should be capable in adjusting their procedures to the particular requirements of pediatric patients, cultivating a positive and agreeable climate during circulatory strain evaluations.

6. **Moves in Teenagers and Change to Grown-up Care:**
Checking pulse in youths includes exceptional difficulties connected with the physiological changes related with adolescence, way of life factors,

and the progress from pediatric to grown-up care. Young people might encounter vacillations in circulatory strain because of hormonal changes, expanded independence in way of life decisions, and likely commitment to hazardous ways of behaving. The progress to grown-up care requires a consistent handover of obligation from pediatric to grown-up medical services suppliers. Guaranteeing progression in circulatory strain observing during this change is basic for tending to arising cardiovascular gamble factors and keeping up with ideal long haul wellbeing results.

7. **Innovative Contemplations and Hardware Choice:**
The decision of circulatory strain estimation hardware and the combination of innovation represent extra difficulties in pediatric settings. Pediatric patients might be more delicate to the customary inflatable sleeves utilized in computerized pulse screens. Choosing properly estimated sleeves for various age bunches is fundamental to acquire precise readings.

Mechanical headways, including oscillometric gadgets and wearable screens, offer options for pulse observing in pediatric patients. Notwithstanding, the approval and exactness of these advances in different pediatric populaces require continuous exploration and normalization to guarantee dependable estimations.

8. **The Job of Parental Contribution and Home Checking:**
Parental contribution is vital to the effective observing of pulse in pediatric patients, particularly with regards to home checking. Instructing guardians about the significance of normal circulatory strain estimations at home, legitimate procedure, and the meaning of keeping a pulse log improves the general administration of pediatric hypertension. Home checking gives a more thorough image of a kid's pulse profile, supports the recognizable proof of white coat hypertension, and works with progressing correspondence among guardians and medical services suppliers.

9. **Challenges in Youngsters with Unique Medical services Needs:**
Kids with exceptional medical care needs, incorporating those with ongoing ailments or formative handicaps, present one of a kind difficulties in pulse observing. These difficulties might come from challenges in correspondence, social contemplations, or the presence of comorbidities that effect pulse guideline. Medical services suppliers should take on individualized approaches, team up with multidisciplinary groups, and influence elective observing techniques to guarantee precise and dependable pulse estimations in this assorted patient populace.

10. **Social Awareness and Correspondence Difficulties:**
Social variables and correspondence difficulties can impact the exactness of circulatory strain checking in pediatric patients. Successful correspondence with youngsters and their families, considering social standards,

convictions, and language inclinations, is fundamental for building trust and working with precise estimations. Medical services suppliers ought to be receptive to social responsive qualities that might influence the youngster's solace and collaboration during circulatory strain evaluations, guaranteeing a socially capable way to deal with pediatric consideration.

11. **Tending to Uneasiness and Stress in Pediatric Patients:**
Uneasiness and stress assume a critical part in pulse estimations, particularly in pediatric patients. The trepidation or inconvenience related with clinical settings can add to raised readings, prompting potential misdiagnosis of hypertension. Youngster cordial conditions, age-proper correspondence, and procedures to lighten uneasiness add to a more informal environment for circulatory strain checking. Medical care suppliers ought to utilize youngster life subject matter experts or other help faculty to make a positive encounter and moderate pressure during pulse evaluations.

12. **Instruction and Preparing for Medical services Suppliers:**

Guaranteeing precise pulse checking in pediatric patients requires progressing schooling and preparing for medical care suppliers. Pediatricians, nurture, and associated wellbeing experts should keep up to date with refreshed rules, development diagrams, and regulating information intended for pediatric populaces. Preparing projects ought to underline the subtleties of circulatory strain estimation methods, the choice of suitable hardware, and the translation of results. Consistent expert improvement guarantees that medical care suppliers are exceptional to explore the intricacies of circulatory strain observing in pediatric patients.

6.3 Success Stories in Hypertension Management

Examples of overcoming adversity in hypertension the board mirror the extraordinary effect of extensive and cooperative ways to deal with care. Hypertension, frequently alluded to as the "quiet executioner," is a constant condition that, when left uncontrolled, presents critical dangers to cardiovascular wellbeing. The examples of overcoming adversity introduced here feature the accomplishments in hypertension the executives, going from way of life changes and creative mediations to patient schooling and local area based drives. These accounts highlight the significance of early discovery, customized care, and the aggregate endeavors of medical services suppliers, people, and networks.

1. **Customized Way of life Alterations:**
An example of overcoming adversity in hypertension the board frequently starts with customized way of life changes. One such story includes a

moderately aged individual determined to have hypertension during a standard exam. Rather than promptly depending on meds, the medical services supplier teamed up with the patient to foster a customized plan that included dietary changes, expanded active work, and stress decrease procedures. The patient focused on making economical way of life alterations, for example, embracing the Scramble (Dietary Ways to deal with Stop Hypertension) diet, taking part in standard activity, and rehearsing care. Over the long haul, the patient accomplished critical pulse decreases, featuring the force of customized, patient-focused approaches in overseeing hypertension.

2. **Local area Based Pulse Observing Projects:**
   Progress in hypertension the executives stretches out past individual cases to local area wide drives. Locally where hypertension pervasiveness was high, a medical care association carried out a local area based pulse checking program. This drive included setting up circulatory strain checking stations at nearby drug stores, public venues, and public spaces. Prepared volunteers instructed local area individuals about the significance of standard circulatory strain checks and gave assets on solid living. The program worked with early location of hypertension as well as enabled people to assume command over their wellbeing. Thus, the local area saw a remarkable decrease in normal pulse levels over the long haul.

3. **Telehealth and Remote Observing:**
   The coming of telehealth and remote observing advances has upset hypertension the executives, especially with regards to the continuous worldwide shift towards virtual medical care. An example of overcoming adversity includes a country local area where admittance to specific medical services was restricted. Through telehealth stages, people with hypertension got virtual conferences, empowering medical care suppliers to screen circulatory strain from a distance. Furthermore, wearable gadgets permitted constant following of pulse levels, giving ongoing information to medical care experts. This approach further developed openness to mind as well as engaged people to partake in their hypertension the executives, cultivating a feeling of control and responsibility effectively.

4. **Multidisciplinary Care Groups:**
   Progress in hypertension the executives frequently includes the cooperation of multidisciplinary care groups. For a situation where a patient had numerous persistent circumstances, including hypertension, a consideration group comprising of essential consideration doctors, cardiologists, dietitians, and conduct wellbeing experts cooperated. The group fostered a coordinated consideration plan that tended to pulse control as well as the interconnected parts of the patient's wellbeing. Standard group gatherings worked with correspondence and acclimations to the consideration

plan, prompting worked on understanding results. The progress in over-seeing hypertension was essential for a more extensive way to deal with comprehensive medical care.

5. **Patient Training and Strengthening:**
Enabling people with hypertension through training is a foundation of examples of overcoming adversity in administration. In a patient schooling drive, people went to studios where medical care experts gave data on hypertension, its ramifications, and commonsense systems for self-administration. Patients found out about drug adherence, the significance of checking circulatory strain at home, and the job of way of life adjustments. This training expanded mindfulness as well as enabled people to take part in their consideration effectively. The achievement was clear as members showed further developed pulse control and a feeling of trust in dealing with their condition.

6. **Inventive Prescription Adherence Projects:**
Drug adherence is a basic calculate hypertension the board, and examples of overcoming adversity feature inventive projects intended to upgrade adherence. In one program, a medical care framework utilized versatile applications and brilliant pill gadgets to help prescription adherence among patients with hypertension. The application sent updates for medicine consumption, followed adherence, and gave instructive assets. The savvy pill container, furnished with sensors, guaranteed that portions were taken at the recommended times. This blend of innovation and patient commitment prompted eminent enhancements in prescription adherence and ensuing circulatory strain control.

7. **Working environment Wellbeing Projects:**
Working environment wellbeing drives have arisen as effective roads for overseeing hypertension, perceiving the effect of way of life factors in an individual's day to day climate. In a corporate setting, a far reaching work environment wellbeing program was carried out, including wellness classes, good dieting choices in the cafeteria, and stress the executives studios. Ordinary circulatory strain registers were coordinated with yearly wellbeing screenings. Thus, representatives experienced upgrades in by and large wellbeing, with a huge decrease in the commonness of hypertension among the labor force. The progress of the program helped individual representatives as well as added to a better work environment culture.

8. **Socially Custom fitted Methodologies:**
Perceiving the different social foundations of people is necessary to fruitful hypertension the executives. An example of overcoming adversity includes a medical care association that carried out socially fitted ways to deal with address hypertension inside unambiguous ethnic networks.

Local area wellbeing laborers conversant in the particular dialects and acquainted with social subtleties led outreach programs. The materials and assets were adjusted to line up with social inclinations, guaranteeing importance and reverberation. This approach prompted expanded commitment, better comprehension of hypertension, and further developed adherence to way of life changes and treatment plans inside these networks.

9. **Pediatric Hypertension Anticipation Projects:**
   Progress in hypertension the board likewise reaches out to preventive endeavors, particularly in pediatric populaces. A pediatric medical care framework executed a thorough counteraction program in schools, underscoring the significance of a solid way of life since the beginning. The program included nourishment training, actual work drives, and routine circulatory strain screenings for young kids. By imparting sound propensities from the beginning, the program added to a decrease in the predominance of life as a youngster hypertension, establishing the groundwork for a better adulthood.

10. **Patient Care Groups:**
    Patient care groups assume an essential part in encouraging a feeling of local area, shared encounters, and everyday encouragement among people overseeing hypertension. In one example of overcoming adversity, a patient care group gave a stage to people with hypertension to associate, share difficulties, and celebrate triumphs. The gathering offered instructive meetings, worked with by medical care experts, on points going from drug the board to pressure decrease procedures. The kinship and common help inside the gathering added to further developed adherence, better circulatory strain control, and improved by and large prosperity.

11. **Strategy Backing for Hypertension Mindfulness:**
    Examples of overcoming adversity in hypertension the executives frequently include backing at the strategy level to bring issues to light and drive foundational change.
    An alliance of medical care experts, patient backers, and policymakers teamed up to advocate for expanded hypertension mindfulness and preventive measures. This promotion prompted the execution of general wellbeing efforts, strategy changes in school educational programs to incorporate hypertension training, and further developed admittance to reasonable, nutritious food choices in underserved networks. These strategy driven drives added to a positive change in local area wellbeing results.

12. **Longitudinal Consideration and Consistent Observing:**

Outcome in hypertension the board is certainly not a one-time accomplishment yet a constant cycle that requires longitudinal consideration and checking. In a fruitful case, a medical services framework carried out a non-stop consideration model, guaranteeing that people with hypertension got progressing support, customary subsequent meet-ups, and changes in accordance with their consideration plans depending on the situation. Persistent observing, including telehealth registrations and standard circulatory strain appraisals, permitted medical services suppliers to proactively address changes in wellbeing status and upgrade the board systems over the long haul.

CHAPTER 7

Nutrition and Growth in Pediatric Nephrology

Sustenance and development are basic parts of pediatric nephrology, assuming an essential part in the general wellbeing and prosperity of youngsters with kidney-related conditions. The transaction between sustenance, development, and kidney capability is many-sided, and dealing with these viewpoints turns out to be much more essential when youngsters face difficulties connected with renal problems. This investigation dives into the complicated connection among sustenance and development in pediatric nephrology, enveloping the effect of renal problems on healthful status, the job of diet in overseeing kidney conditions, development contemplations, and the multidisciplinary approach expected to upgrade the wholesome prosperity of youngsters with kidney-related issues.

1. **Effect of Renal Issues on Wholesome Status:**
   Youngsters with kidney issues frequently face critical difficulties in keeping up with ideal nourishing status. The kidneys assume a focal part in directing liquid and electrolyte balance, discharging side-effects, and blending chemicals engaged with bone wellbeing and red platelet creation.

   At the point when kidney capability is compromised, as found in conditions like constant kidney illness (CKD) or nephrotic disorder, these administrative capabilities are disabled. Youngsters with CKD, for instance, may encounter modified digestion, protein-energy squandering, and challenges in keeping up with satisfactory development. Nephrotic disorder, described by proteinuria and hypoalbuminemia, further worsens the gamble of unhealthiness. The effect of renal problems on wholesome status requires fitted dietary intercessions to address explicit necessities and difficulties.

2. **Job of Diet in Overseeing Kidney Conditions:**
Dietary administration is a foundation being taken care of by youngsters with kidney conditions. Contingent upon the particular renal issue, dietary suggestions might differ, however shared objectives incorporate controlling protein admission, overseeing liquid and electrolyte balance, and tending to explicit supplement needs. In CKD, for example, there is much of the time a need to limit dietary phosphorus and potassium, as weakened kidney capability influences their discharge. Sodium limitation might be important to oversee liquid equilibrium and pulse. Satisfactory protein admission is fundamental, yet its amount might be changed in view of the phase of CKD. In nephrotic condition, where protein misfortune through pee is a worry, dietary protein might should be expanded to make up for misfortunes. The cautious administration of these dietary parts is imperative to help kidney capability and relieve entanglements.

3. **Development Contemplations in Pediatric Nephrology:**
Ideal development is a critical sign of in general wellbeing in kids, and its assessment becomes vital with regards to pediatric nephrology. Youngsters with kidney problems might confront development challenges because of elements like impeded supplement assimilation, metabolic anomalies, hormonal unsettling influences, and the effect of persistent sicknesses. Hindered development, deferred pubescence, and diminished last grown-up level are likely worries. The evaluation of development includes following level, weight, and weight file (BMI) after some time, taking into account age and orientation explicit development graphs. Medical care suppliers in pediatric nephrology cautiously screen development boundaries to recognize deviations and mediate immediately with customized dietary procedures and clinical intercessions.

4. **Protein-Energy Squandering and Ailing health:**
Protein-energy squandering (Seat) is a predominant entanglement in pediatric nephrology, especially in youngsters with cutting edge CKD. Seat includes the deficiency of body protein and energy stores, prompting muscle squandering, decreased strength, and compromised invulnerable capability. Ailing health, portrayed by deficient admission of fundamental supplements, intensifies the gamble of Seat. Youngsters with kidney issues might encounter unfortunate craving, dietary limitations, and changed taste insights, further adding to unhealthiness.
The administration of Seat and hunger includes enhancing protein and caloric admission, tending to explicit supplement inadequacies, and taking into account nourishing supplementation when important. The objective is to help development, keep up with bulk, and improve generally speaking prosperity.

5. **Liquid and Electrolyte The board:**
   Liquid and electrolyte balance is unpredictably connected to renal capability, and disturbances in this equilibrium can significantly affect the soundness of youngsters with kidney problems. Conditions, for example, CKD might bring about debilitated liquid discharge, prompting liquid maintenance and electrolyte awkward nature. Sodium and potassium are basic electrolytes that require cautious observing with regards to pediatric nephrology. Dietary mediations, like limiting sodium and potassium consumption, become fundamental in dealing with these irregular characteristics. Liquid limitation might be important in specific cases to forestall volume over-burden. Adjusting these dietary parts is vital to forestall entanglements like hypertension, edema, and electrolyte unsettling influences.

6. **Job of Micronutrients:**
   Micronutrients, including nutrients and minerals, assume a urgent part in supporting different physiological capabilities, and their administration becomes critical in pediatric nephrology. Youngsters with kidney issues might be in danger of micronutrient lacks because of variables like dietary limitations, impeded assimilation, or expanded misfortunes. For instance, vitamin D lack is normal in CKD, affecting bone wellbeing. Lack of iron might happen in conditions related with sickliness. Observing and tending to these micronutrient needs are imperative for generally speaking wellbeing and may include dietary adjustments, oral enhancements, or intravenous supplementation when important.

7. **Multidisciplinary Way to deal with Dietary Consideration:**
   Streamlining sustenance in pediatric nephrology requires a multidisciplinary approach that includes coordinated effort among medical services experts, including pediatric nephrologists, dietitians, medical attendants, and different trained professionals. Dietitians assume a focal part in planning individualized dietary plans, taking into account the particular requirements and limitations related with various renal problems. Standard appraisals, including anthropometric estimations, research facility tests, and development observing, guide changes in accordance with the wholesome consideration plan. The cooperative endeavors of the medical care group guarantee an all encompassing way to deal with dealing with the wholesome prosperity of youngsters with kidney-related conditions.

8. **Challenges in Healthful Administration:**
   Notwithstanding the significance of nourishing administration in pediatric nephrology, a few difficulties exist. Dietary limitations, especially in conditions like CKD, may prompt restricted food decisions and decreased tastefulness, influencing adherence to dietary suggestions.
   Youngsters might encounter unfortunate craving or repugnances for

specific food varieties. Furthermore, the effect of constant sickness on the psychosocial parts of eating ought not be disregarded. Adherence to dietary plans might be impacted by variables like relational intricacies, financial status, and social inclinations. Beating these difficulties requires continuous correspondence, schooling, and backing from the medical care group.

9. **Dietary Help and Supplementation:**
In situations where dietary mediations alone may not address healthful issues, or when oral admission is compromised, nourishing help and supplementation become fundamental. Enteral sustenance, conveyed through tube taking care of, might be considered for youngsters with critical hunger or troubles in oral admission. Particular nourishing equations custom fitted to the particular necessities of pediatric nephrology are accessible. Intravenous nourishment might be vital in extreme situations where oral or enteral courses are not practical. The objective of healthful help is to guarantee that youngsters get sufficient supplements for development, improvement, and in general prosperity.

10. **Long haul Effect on Personal satisfaction:**
The drawn out effect of wholesome administration in pediatric nephrology stretches out past prompt wellbeing results and envelops the general personal satisfaction for youngsters and their families. Very much oversaw sustenance adds to better development, diminished intricacies, and further developed energy levels. By tending to dietary necessities, medical services suppliers plan to improve the general prosperity of kids, permitting them to participate in age-suitable exercises, go to class, and take part in friendly collaborations. Guaranteeing ideal sustenance is a major part of encouraging a positive and satisfying personal satisfaction for youngsters with kidney-related conditions.

11. **Change to Grown-up Care:**

As youngsters with kidney problems progress to adulthood, the congruity of dietary consideration turns into a basic thought. The progress from pediatric to grown-up nephrology care includes tending to advancing healthful requirements, adjusting dietary plans, and enabling youthful grown-ups to play a functioning job in dealing with their sustenance. The coordinated effort among pediatric and grown-up medical services groups guarantees a consistent change, with an emphasis on keeping up with wholesome prosperity all through the existence course.

7.1 Nutritional Challenges in Pediatric Kidney Patients

Nourishing difficulties in pediatric kidney patients present a perplexing scene that requires a customized and multidisciplinary approach. Youngsters with kidney problems face special dietary contemplations because of the mind boggling connection between kidney capability, development, and by and large prosperity.

This investigation dives into the particular healthful difficulties experienced by pediatric kidney patients, including issues connected with protein and calorie the board, liquid and electrolyte balance, micronutrient lacks, development contemplations, and the effect of constant kidney infections (CKD) and other renal problems on the dietary status of youngsters.

1. **Protein and Calorie The executives:**
   Protein and calorie the board is a focal part of the wholesome difficulties looked by pediatric kidney patients. In conditions like CKD, there is a fragile harmony between giving satisfactory supplements to development and improvement and staying away from extreme protein consumption that can strain compromised kidneys. Protein limitation is in many cases important to oversee uremic side effects and forestall protein-energy squandering. In any case, deficient protein admission can prompt development hindrance and nourishing lacks. Adjusting calorie admission is similarly essential, as youngsters with kidney problems might have expanded energy needs because of the requests of their ailment. Dietary techniques should cautiously address both protein and calorie the board, meaning to advance development while supporting kidney capability.

2. **Liquid and Electrolyte Equilibrium:**
   Keeping up with liquid and electrolyte balance is a huge test in pediatric kidney patients, especially those with disabled renal capability. The kidneys assume an imperative part in controlling liquid volume and electrolyte fixations in the body. In CKD, the capacity to discharge abundance liquids and keep up with electrolyte balance is compromised. Sodium and potassium limitations are normal dietary intercessions to forestall liquid maintenance, hypertension, and electrolyte uneven characters. Nonetheless, severe liquid limitations can affect youngsters' hydration status, prompting difficulties in gathering their general liquid requirements. Exploring the fragile harmony between liquid and electrolyte the board is significant for forestalling complexities while guaranteeing satisfactory hydration and supplement admission.

3. **Micronutrient Inadequacies:**
   Micronutrient lacks represent a critical nourishing test in pediatric kidney patients. Conditions like CKD can upset the equilibrium between fundamental nutrients and minerals, prompting lacks that influence generally speaking wellbeing. Normal micronutrient concerns remember lacks for vitamin D, calcium, iron, and folic corrosive. Lack of vitamin D, specifically, is pervasive in CKD and adds to bone anomalies and weakened

development. Lack of iron might result from diminished erythropoietin creation, prompting frailty. Tending to these micronutrient lacks requires designated supplementation, dietary alterations, and ordinary checking to forestall long haul entanglements.

4. **Development Contemplations:**

   Ideal development is a critical sign of by and large wellbeing in youngsters, and development contemplations become vital with regards to pediatric kidney patients. Kids with CKD frequently face difficulties connected with development impedance, postponed pubescence, and diminished last grown-up level. Factors adding to development issues incorporate hormonal unsettling influences, metabolic anomalies, and the effect of constant sicknesses. Checking development boundaries, including level, weight, and BMI, is fundamental for recognizing deviations and executing ideal intercessions. Nourishment assumes a focal part in supporting development, and dietary techniques should be customized to address the particular necessities of pediatric kidney patients to relieve the gamble of hindered development.

5. **Effect of Constant Kidney Sicknesses:**

   Constant kidney sicknesses (CKD) fundamentally influence the wholesome status of pediatric patients, presenting a horde of difficulties. CKD is portrayed by the dynamic loss of kidney capability over the long haul, prompting a scope of metabolic and physiological unsettling influences. In the beginning phases of CKD, dietary alterations frequently center around protein and phosphorus limitation to oversee uremic side effects and forestall entanglements. As CKD advances, dietary difficulties heighten, including the requirement for cautious administration of liquid equilibrium, electrolytes, and corrosive base status. Kids with CKD are in danger of protein-energy squandering, hunger, and difficulties like renal osteodystrophy. The powerful idea of CKD requires continuous acclimations to dietary intends to address advancing healthful necessities and forestall antagonistic results.

6. **Liquid Admission Limitations:**

   Pediatric kidney patients, particularly those with cutting edge CKD, may confront liquid admission limitations as a component of their dietary administration. Liquid limitations are executed to forestall volume overburden, hypertension, and electrolyte uneven characters. In any case, restricting liquid admission can be trying for kids, influencing their general hydration status and influencing everyday exercises. The fragile harmony between forestalling complexities related with liquid over-burden and guaranteeing satisfactory hydration is a steady test in the nourishing consideration of pediatric kidney patients. Medical services suppliers should work cooperatively with families to foster methodologies that address liquid limitations while supporting youngsters' prosperity.

7. **Healthful Help and Enteral Sustenance:**
In situations where dietary mediations alone may not meet the nourishing requirements of pediatric kidney patients, wholesome help and enteral sustenance might be thought of. Enteral sustenance includes the conveyance of supplements through a cylinder, addressing difficulties connected with oral admission or gastrointestinal ingestion.

Particular wholesome equations are intended to meet the particular necessities of pediatric patients with kidney problems, giving fundamental supplements in a controlled way. Healthful help assumes an essential part in forestalling lack of healthy sustenance, advancing development, and supporting generally speaking prosperity in circumstances where oral admission is compromised.

8. **Psychosocial and Social Elements:**
The psychosocial and social parts of sustenance present extra difficulties under the watchful eye of pediatric kidney patients. Youngsters might encounter adjusted taste discernments, loss of hunger, or repugnances for explicit food varieties because of the effect of kidney issues. The psychosocial stress related with constant sickness can additionally add to changes in dietary patterns and dietary inclinations. Understanding and addressing these variables are necessary to the outcome of healthful intercessions. Cooperative endeavors including dietitians, clinicians, and medical care suppliers are fundamental in supporting youngsters and their families in exploring the psychosocial aspects of healthful difficulties.

9. **Change to Grown-up Care:**
The change from pediatric to grown-up care adds a layer of intricacy to the nourishing difficulties looked by pediatric kidney patients. As teenagers with kidney problems progress to grown-up nephrology care, there is a need to adjust dietary plans, address developing wholesome necessities, and enable youthful grown-ups to play a functioning job in dealing with their nourishment. The coherence of care during this progress period is urgent to guaranteeing that healthful intercessions stay powerful and customized to the changing necessities of the developing person.

10. **Instructive and Strong Techniques:**

Instructive and strong techniques assume a urgent part in tending to dietary difficulties in pediatric kidney patients. Furnishing families with extensive schooling about dietary changes, liquid limitations, and the significance of healthful help upgrades their capacity to explore the intricacies of dealing with a youngster's nourishing requirements. Steady procedures might incorporate including a multidisciplinary medical care group, offering guiding administrations, and encouraging companion support gatherings to address the psychosocial parts of healthful difficulties. Enabling families with information and backing adds to further developed adherence to dietary plans and upgrades the general personal satisfaction for pediatric kidney patients.

7.2 Triumphs in Optimizing Growth and Development

Wins in advancing development and improvement in pediatric nephrology address critical achievements that mirror the progress of extensive and co-operative medical services draws near. Youngsters with kidney-related conditions face special difficulties that can influence their development directions and by and large turn of events.

This investigation digs into the victories accomplished in the domain of pediatric nephrology, featuring examples of overcoming adversity, creative mediations, and multidisciplinary endeavors that have added to the better development and improvement of youngsters confronting kidney-related difficulties.

1. **Customized Development Checking and Mediation:**
   One victory in advancing development and advancement includes the execution of customized development checking and mediation plans. Pediatric nephrology groups, in a joint effort with dietitians and other medical care experts, have created fitted systems to screen and address individual development concerns. By utilizing standard appraisals of level, weight, and weight file (BMI) alongside age-explicit development graphs, medical services suppliers can distinguish deviations and intercede quickly. Customized development plans might incorporate nourishing changes, hormonal intercessions, and psychosocial backing to address the special requirements of every youngster. These customized approaches have brought about better development results, displaying the adequacy of designated intercessions.

2. **Imaginative Healthful Methodologies:**
   Advancement in healthful methodologies plays had a critical impact in wins connected with development and improvement in pediatric nephrology. Dietitians and nutritionists team up to plan creative dietary plans that balance the healthful necessities of youngsters with kidney-related conditions. This incorporates individualized ways to deal with protein and calorie the executives, micronutrient supplementation, and specific healthful equations. Developments in enteral nourishment, for example, tube taking care of with modified equations, have given a reasonable answer for kids confronting difficulties with oral admission. These creative

dietary procedures have streamlined development as well as improved the generally wholesome prosperity of pediatric patients.

3. **Progressions in Hormonal Treatments:**
Progressions in hormonal treatments have contributed altogether to wins in upgrading development and advancement in youngsters with kidney issues. Development chemical treatment, for example, has been effectively utilized to address development disability related with constant kidney illnesses (CKD). By animating direct development, development chemical treatment has demonstrated viable in working on conclusive grown-up level in youngsters with CKD. This win features how designated hormonal mediations can alleviate the effect of renal problems on development and improvement, permitting youngsters to accomplish their full development potential.

4. **Multidisciplinary Care Groups:**
The foundation of multidisciplinary care groups addresses a victory in pediatric nephrology, especially concerning development and improvement.

These groups ordinarily incorporate pediatric nephrologists, dietitians, endocrinologists, analysts, and different experts working cooperatively to address the assorted necessities of youngsters with kidney-related conditions. The all encompassing methodology of multidisciplinary care perceives the interconnected idea of development and improvement, tending to the physiological viewpoints as well as the psychosocial aspects. This cooperative model has demonstrated compelling in fitting mediations, giving far reaching care, and accomplishing positive results in advancing development and advancement.

5. **Psychosocial Backing Drives:**
Wins in enhancing development and improvement stretch out past physiological mediations to envelop psychosocial support drives. The close to home and mental prosperity of pediatric patients assumes a significant part in their general turn of events. Clinicians and social specialists work together with medical care groups to carry out help programs, directing administrations, and friend support gatherings. These drives assist youngsters and their families with adapting to the difficulties of kidney-related conditions, lessening pressure and nervousness that might affect development. The victories in psychosocial support add to an all encompassing methodology that tends to both the physical and close to home parts of pediatric nephrology care.

6. **Change Projects for Young people:**
Change programs intended for young people progressing from pediatric to grown-up nephrology care address a victory in coherence of care. Guaranteeing a smooth progress is fundamental for keeping up with

development and improvement directions as youngsters enter adulthood. Progress programs include instructive drives, advising meetings, and co-operative endeavors among pediatric and grown-up medical care groups. By planning youths for the progressions in medical care the executives, nourishing necessities, and psychosocial contemplations, these projects add to positive results in development and improvement during the basic time of change.

7. **Patient and Family Training:**
Wins in development and improvement streamlining are intently attached to patient and family training drives. Giving complete training about the idea of kidney-related conditions, the significance of adherence to treatment plans, and the job of nourishment in development has enabled families to take part under the watchful eye of their youngsters effectively. Grasping the effect of adherence to meds, dietary suggestions, and way of life alterations has prompted superior consistence and improved results in development and advancement. Schooling fills in as an incredible asset in encouraging a cooperative organization between medical services suppliers and families.

8. **Telehealth and Remote Observing:**
The combination of telehealth and remote observing advancements has arisen as a victory in improving development and improvement, particularly with regards to continuous worldwide movements towards virtual medical services. Telehealth stages permit medical services suppliers to direct virtual interviews, screen development boundaries, and evaluate therapy adherence from a distance. Remote observing gadgets and wearable advances empower consistent following of development related measurements, giving constant information to medical services experts. These advancements upgrade availability to mind, work with ideal intercessions, and add to positive development results for pediatric patients.

9. **Backing for Pediatric Nephrology Exploration:**
Wins in streamlining development and improvement are intently attached to continuous exploration and promotion endeavors in the field of pediatric nephrology. Research drives zeroed in on understanding the basic components of development disability in kidney-related conditions, assessing the viability of mediations, and distinguishing novel restorative methodologies add to headways in care. Backing for expanded financing and backing for pediatric nephrology research guarantees that the field keeps on advancing, prompting inventive methodologies and further developed results for youngsters confronting development and advancement challenges.

10. **Examples of overcoming adversity in Progressed Grown-ups:**
Examples of overcoming adversity including people who progressed from

pediatric nephrology care to grown-up care and accomplished positive development results feature the victories in congruity of care. These examples of overcoming adversity underscore the significance of consistent changes, progressing support, and cooperative endeavors between medical services groups. People who effectively explore the change exhibit that development and improvement advancement is feasible across the life expectancy, supporting the effect of complete and all around facilitated care.

11. **Personal satisfaction Contemplations:**

Wins in upgrading development and improvement line up with a more extensive spotlight on personal satisfaction contemplations for pediatric patients with kidney-related conditions. The combination of methodologies to upgrade generally prosperity, including actual wellbeing, profound wellbeing, and social commitment, adds to positive development results. Personal satisfaction contemplations perceive that development and improvement are not secluded results but rather necessary parts of a youngster's general educational experience. Wins in this domain include a comprehensive methodology that focuses on the youngster's satisfaction, satisfaction, and capacity to participate in age-fitting exercises.

7.3 Multidisciplinary Approaches to Nutrition Management

Multidisciplinary ways to deal with sustenance the executives address an exhaustive and cooperative methodology pointed toward tending to the different dietary necessities of people across different medical services settings. This approach perceives that sustenance is an intricate exchange of physiological, mental, and social variables, requiring the skill of different medical services experts. This investigation digs into the meaning of multidisciplinary ways to deal with nourishment the board, looking at their application in persistent ailments, pediatric consideration, dietary problems, and the maturing populace.

1. **Persistent Ailments and Nourishment:**
   Multidisciplinary ways to deal with sustenance the executives assume a vital part in tending to the complex healthful difficulties related with ongoing sicknesses. Conditions like diabetes, cardiovascular sicknesses, and ongoing kidney illnesses require customized dietary intercessions to oversee side effects, forestall entanglements, and work on by and large prosperity. In these cases, a multidisciplinary group might incorporate dietitians, endocrinologists, cardiologists, nephrologists, and clinicians. Dietitians team up with clinical experts to configuration individualized dietary plans that consider the particular healthful requirements and limitations related with each ongoing ailment. Endocrinologists and

cardiologists give clinical bits of knowledge, guaranteeing that dietary mediations line up with in general treatment objectives. Analysts add to tending to the psychosocial parts of dietary administration, perceiving the effect of constant sicknesses on psychological well-being and way of life ways of behaving. This cooperative model upgrades the viability of wholesome mediations and encourages a comprehensive way to deal with overseeing constant sicknesses.

2. **Pediatric Sustenance Care:**

In the domain of pediatric nourishment, multidisciplinary approaches are instrumental in tending to the special wholesome requirements of youngsters across different medical issue. Pediatric nourishment care groups ordinarily incorporate pediatricians, dietitians, pediatric gastroenterologists, language teachers, and word related advisors. This cooperative methodology is especially obvious in instances of pediatric taking care of problems, where youngsters might confront difficulties connected with oral coordinated movements, tangible issues, or gastrointestinal circumstances. Language instructors evaluate and address gulping hardships, word related specialists take care of on tactile problems affecting taking care of, and dietitians plan sustenance designs that oblige these difficulties. Pediatricians give clinical oversight and direction care, guaranteeing that the kid's dietary requirements line up with generally wellbeing objectives. The outcome of multidisciplinary pediatric nourishment care lies in its capacity to address a range of issues, cultivating ideal development and improvement in kids.

3. **Dietary problems and Wholesome Restoration:**

Multidisciplinary approaches are fundamental in the wholesome recovery of people with dietary issues, for example, anorexia nervosa, bulimia nervosa, and gorging jumble. Dietary problems include complex connections between physiological, mental, and conduct factors, requiring an extensive group of medical services experts. An ordinary dietary problem treatment group might incorporate specialists, clinicians, dietitians, doctors, and medical caretakers. Specialists and clinicians address the mental parts of dietary problems, including misshaped self-perception and scattered eating ways of behaving. Dietitians assume an essential part in wholesome recovery, working intimately with people to lay out smart dieting designs and standardize eating ways of behaving. Doctors and attendants screen actual wellbeing, tending to unexpected issues coming about because of lack of healthy sustenance. This multidisciplinary approach gives all encompassing consideration, tending to both the physical and mental elements of dietary problems, and works with the excursion to healthful recuperation.

4. **Maturing Populace and Healthful Wellbeing:**
   As the worldwide populace ages, the meaning of multidisciplinary ways to deal with wholesome health in the old turns out to be progressively evident. More established grown-ups frequently face one of a kind nourishing difficulties, including diminished hunger, changed supplement ingestion, and persistent diseases. Multidisciplinary groups for geriatric sustenance might include geriatricians, dietitians, medical caretakers, actual advisors, and drug specialists. Geriatricians evaluate by and large wellbeing and address clinical worries, while dietitians tailor nourishment intends to oblige age-related changes and explicit ailments. Attendants offer help for day to day nourishing necessities and screen changes in wellbeing status. Actual specialists add to keeping up with versatility and utilitarian freedom, which is necessary to nourishing health. Drug specialists audit meds that might affect wholesome status and work together with the group to limit unfavorable impacts. The multidisciplinary way to deal with geriatric nourishment perceives the intricacy of elements affecting wholesome health in more seasoned grown-ups and expects to improve their dietary status for upgraded by and large prosperity.

5. **Sports Sustenance and Execution Enhancement:**
   In the domain of sports nourishment, multidisciplinary approaches are utilized to streamline execution, improve recuperation, and forestall wounds. Sports nourishment groups frequently incorporate enlisted dietitians, sports medication doctors, physiologists, and athletic coaches. Enrolled dietitians have some expertise in planning sustenance designs that meet the particular energy and supplement necessities of competitors in light of their game, preparing routine, and individual requirements. Sports medication doctors survey generally wellbeing, address clinical worries, and team up with dietitians to improve nourishing methodologies. Physiologists contribute experiences into the physiological requests of various games, directing nourishment mediations for maximized operation. Athletic mentors offer help for injury anticipation and recuperation, perceiving the job of sustenance in outer muscle wellbeing. This multidisciplinary coordinated effort plans to augment the advantages of sustenance in sports, adding to worked on athletic execution and in general prosperity.

6. **Disease Nourishment Care:**
   Malignant growth sustenance care includes multidisciplinary approaches that address the nourishing difficulties looked by people going through disease treatment. The malignant growth nourishment care group might incorporate oncologists, enrolled dietitians, oncology attendants, and social laborers. Oncologists give clinical oversight and direction malignant growth treatment, while enlisted dietitians foster nourishment designs

that help the wholesome necessities of people during treatment. Oncology medical caretakers assume a urgent part in checking healthful status, overseeing therapy related secondary effects, and giving steady consideration. Social specialists address psychosocial viewpoints, offering directing and backing to people and their families exploring the difficulties of malignant growth treatment. This cooperative model guarantees that dietary intercessions line up with generally malignant growth care, advancing prosperity and versatility during treatment.

7. **Neurological Problems and Sustenance:**
Neurological problems, like Parkinson's illness, numerous sclerosis, and epilepsy, require particular sustenance care that incorporates different medical services disciplines. A multidisciplinary group might incorporate nervous system specialists, enrolled dietitians, actual advisors, and language teachers. Nervous system specialists give clinical aptitude, tending to the neurological parts of the condition and its effect on nourishing prosperity. Enlisted dietitians plan sustenance designs that consider the particular difficulties related with neurological problems, for example, dysphagia or engine hindrances influencing taking care of. Actual specialists center around keeping up with portability and tending to engine capability, which is fundamental to guaranteeing ideal sustenance. Language teachers survey and address gulping hardships, improving nourishing admission. The cooperation of these medical care experts brings about an all encompassing way to deal with overseeing wholesome difficulties in people with neurological problems.

8. **Emotional well-being and Wholesome Psychiatry:**
The arising field of wholesome psychiatry features the interconnectedness of sustenance and psychological wellness, stressing the job of diet in state of mind problems and mental prosperity. Multidisciplinary approaches in wholesome psychiatry include coordinated effort between specialists, dietitians, therapists, and other emotional wellness experts. Specialists give bits of knowledge into the mental parts of emotional wellness conditions and meds that might affect dietary status. Dietitians foster dietary mediations that line up with the standards of healthful psychiatry, underlining the job of specific supplements in supporting mental prosperity. Analysts address the mental parts of eating ways of behaving, stress the board, and close to home prosperity, perceiving the bidirectional connection among sustenance and emotional wellness. This multidisciplinary approach adds to a thorough comprehension of the effect of nourishment on emotional well-being and works with incorporated care for people with emotional well-being conditions.

9. **Innovation Coordination in Nourishment The board:**
The coordination of innovation has additionally improved the adequacy

of multidisciplinary ways to deal with sustenance the board. Electronic wellbeing records (EHRs), telehealth stages, and nourishment applications empower consistent correspondence and joint effort among medical services experts, working with continuous data sharing and facilitated care. Telehealth counsels give remote admittance to dietitians, permitting people to get master wholesome direction without geological requirements. Nourishment applications help people in following dietary propensities, checking wholesome admission, and getting customized suggestions. Innovation combination upholds multidisciplinary groups in conveying productive, patient-focused care, upgrading the openness and viability of nourishment the executives across assorted medical services settings.

10. **Local area Based Sustenance Projects:**

Multidisciplinary approaches reach out past clinical settings to local area based nourishment programs that intend to advance populace wide healthful prosperity. These projects frequently include joint effort between general wellbeing experts, dietitians, local area coordinators, and nearby medical services suppliers. General wellbeing experts evaluate the dietary necessities of the local area, recognize wellbeing incongruities, and plan mediations that address explicit nourishing difficulties. Dietitians contribute ability in creating instructive materials, leading studios, and offering customized nourishment direction. Local area coordinators work with outreach endeavors, drawing in different local area individuals in nourishment centered drives. Nearby medical care suppliers might partake in wellbeing screenings, offering extra help and assets. Local area based sustenance programs represent the force of multidisciplinary coordinated effort in encouraging positive nourishment results on a more extensive scale.

CHAPTER 8

Psychosocial Aspects of Pediatric Nephrology

The psychosocial parts of pediatric nephrology include an expansive range of profound, conduct, and social contemplations that essentially influence the prosperity of youngsters and their families confronting kidney-related conditions. Exploring the difficulties presented by ongoing sicknesses, renal issues, and the complicated therapy regimens related with pediatric nephrology requires a far reaching comprehension of the psychosocial aspects. This investigation dives into the complex psychosocial parts of pediatric nephrology, tending to the profound effect on youngsters and families, survival techniques, instructive difficulties, and the job of medical services suppliers in cultivating all encompassing consideration.

1. **Close to home Effect on Kids:**
   Youngsters with kidney-related conditions frequently experience a scope of feelings connected with their determination, therapy, and the effect of persistent disease on their regular routines. The close to home effect shifts relying upon variables like the seriousness of the condition, treatment modalities, and the kid's age and formative stage.

   More youthful kids might battle to fathom the intricacies of their clinical circumstance, prompting tension, dread, and disarray. Young people, then again, may wrestle with issues of character, self-perception, and the difficulties of dealing with a persistent sickness during a basic time of self-improvement.

   The profound cost reaches out to worries about peer acknowledgment, expected interruptions to scholarly and social exercises, and the apprehension about operations. Youngsters going through dialysis or transplantation might encounter increased pressure because of the obtrusive idea of these medicines. Medical care suppliers in pediatric nephrology assume a pivotal part in perceiving and tending to these personal difficulties, offering age-suitable help, and encouraging a climate where kids feel open to communicating their sentiments and concerns.

2. **Influence on Relational peculiarities:**
A pediatric nephrology finding resounds through the whole nuclear family, influencing relational peculiarities and connections. Guardians frequently bear the profound weight of dealing with their kid's wellbeing, managing therapy related stressors, and exploring the vulnerabilities related with persistent sickness. Kin might encounter a scope of feelings, including sensations of culpability, stress, or hatred as consideration and assets are redirected towards the youngster with kidney-related conditions.

Family schedules might go through huge changes because of clinical arrangements, dietary limitations, and the requests of therapy regimens. Monetary stressors connected with medical services expenses can additionally strain relational intricacies. Psychosocial support for families in pediatric nephrology includes tending to these difficulties, giving assets to adapting, and empowering open correspondence inside the family. Support gatherings and guiding administrations assume a crucial part in assisting families with exploring the profound intricacies that emerge with regards to pediatric nephrology.

3. **Strategies for dealing with stress:**
Survival strategies are vital for youngsters and families managing the personal difficulties of pediatric nephrology. Versatile survival methods add to strength and the capacity to explore the high points and low points of constant disease. Kids might foster survival techniques, for example, keeping an uplifting perspective, participating in imaginative outlets, or looking for help from companions and friends. Instructive projects and mediations that emphasis on showing kids and their families viable survival methods can improve their capacity to oversee pressure and profound trouble.

For guardians and parental figures, survival strategies might include looking for social help, joining guardian backing gatherings, or getting to directing administrations. Peer encouraging groups of people give an open door to families to associate with others confronting comparative difficulties, share encounters, and trade survival techniques.

Medical care suppliers in pediatric nephrology can effectively advance and work with the improvement of adapting abilities, perceiving the significance of close to home prosperity close by clinical administration.

4. **Instructive Difficulties and School Backing:**
Youngsters with kidney-related conditions might experience instructive difficulties because of unlucky deficiencies connected with clinical arrangements, hospitalizations, or treatment systems. The effect of

persistent disease on a kid's scholarly execution, social communications, and generally speaking school experience requires cooperation between medical services suppliers, instructors, and families. Pediatric nephrology groups can liaise with school work force to make individualized instruction plans (IEPs) that oblige the special necessities of kids with renal issues.

Instructive help might include giving extra assets, changing scholastic assumptions, and guaranteeing that educators are educated about the youngster's ailment. Psychosocial parts of training incorporate tending to likely harassing, encouraging a steady school climate, and advancing mindfulness and understanding among cohorts. School clinicians and guides assume a basic part in supporting the close to home prosperity of youngsters with kidney-related conditions, offering devices to adapt to the difficulties they might look in the instructive setting.

5. **Medical care Supplier Correspondence and Backing:**
Compelling correspondence and backing from medical services suppliers are basic parts of tending to the psychosocial parts of pediatric nephrology. Laying out transparent correspondence channels encourages trust between medical care suppliers, youngsters, and their families. Medical services suppliers should recognize and approve the profound encounters of youngsters and guardians, making a place of refuge for communicating concerns, fears, and vulnerabilities.

Giving far reaching data about the ailment, treatment choices, and potential results enables families to pursue informed choices and effectively partake in the kid's consideration. Psychosocial support administrations, like social work, youngster life subject matter experts, and psychological well-being experts, ought to be coordinated into the pediatric nephrology group. These experts contribute aptitude in tending to close to home necessities, working with survival techniques, and offering direction on exploring the psychosocial intricacies of persistent sickness.

6. **Change to Grown-up Care:**
The change from pediatric to grown-up care is a huge achievement in the excursion of young people with kidney-related conditions. This progress presents extra psychosocial contemplations, including the difficulties of adjusting to another medical services climate, building associations with grown-up medical care suppliers, and getting a sense of ownership with taking care of oneself.

Young people might encounter uneasiness about the vulnerabilities related with changing to another clinical group and adjusting to the grown-up medical services framework.

Psychosocial support during this progress includes getting ready teenagers for the progressions in medical services the executives, giving training on self-promotion, and addressing profound worries connected with the change in care settings. Change programs that work with a steady progress, include both pediatric and grown-up medical care suppliers, and consolidate psychosocial support administrations add to positive results in the profound prosperity of youths exploring this basic stage.

7. **Psychological wellness Screening and Intercession:**
Given the perplexing interchange between ongoing disease and emotional well-being, normal psychological wellness screening and intercession are fundamental parts of pediatric nephrology care. Youngsters and youths with kidney-related conditions might be at an expanded gamble of creating nervousness, misery, or other psychological well-being issues. Routine psychological well-being evaluations permit medical care suppliers to recognize close to home trouble early and execute convenient intercessions.

Coordinated psychological wellness administrations, including advising and psychotherapy, are essential for tending to psychosocial challenges. Emotional well-being experts work together with pediatric nephrology groups to offer help customized to the novel requirements of youngsters and their families. Perceiving and addressing emotional wellness worries close by clinical administration adds to a comprehensive way to deal with pediatric nephrology care, advancing generally speaking prosperity.

8. **Influence on Personal satisfaction:**

The psychosocial parts of pediatric nephrology essentially impact the general personal satisfaction for youngsters and their families. Personal satisfaction contemplations envelop actual wellbeing, close to home prosperity, social cooperations, and the capacity to participate in ordinary exercises. Pediatric nephrology care that focuses on psychosocial support adds to worked on personal satisfaction by tending to profound misery, upgrading survival techniques, and encouraging versatility.

Endeavors to limit the disturbances brought about by constant sickness, for example, integrating play treatment, instructive help, and sporting exercises, add to a more certain personal satisfaction for pediatric patients. Family-focused care that perceives the interconnectedness of clinical and psychosocial viewpoints guarantees an all encompassing way to deal with improving the general prosperity of youngsters confronting kidney-related conditions.

8.1 Impact of Chronic Illness on Pediatric Patients and Families
The effect of constant sickness on pediatric patients and their families is significant, contacting each part of their lives and requiring an intricate and progressing interaction of transformation and strength. Constant sicknesses in youngsters envelop a great many circumstances, from inborn problems to

immune system illnesses, requiring delayed clinical administration and frequently impacting the physical, profound, social, and financial elements of the impacted people and their families. This investigation dives into the multilayered effect of persistent ailment on pediatric patients and families, inspecting the difficulties they face and the methodologies utilized to explore this complex scene.

1. **Actual Wellbeing Difficulties:**
   The actual wellbeing challenges related with persistent ailment in pediatric patients are assorted and can appear in different ways relying upon the idea of the condition. For certain youngsters, the constant ailment might prompt constraints in versatility, ongoing agony, exhaustion, or entanglements influencing numerous organ frameworks. The administration of side effects frequently includes a routine of drugs, operations, and way of life changes that can influence a kid's day to day daily practice and in general prosperity.

   Youngsters with persistent sicknesses might encounter incessant hospitalizations, medical procedures, or extended therapy plans, upsetting their typical exercises and schedules. Adherence to therapy plans, including drug timetables and dietary limitations, becomes critical yet can likewise be requesting for both the youngster and their guardians. Dealing with the actual wellbeing challenges requires a cooperative exertion between medical services suppliers, patients, and families to streamline care and limit the effect on the youngster's everyday existence.

2. **Profound and Mental Effect:**
   The profound and mental effect of persistent disease on pediatric patients is huge and shifts relying upon elements like the seriousness of the condition, the youngster's age, and their survival techniques. Kids might wrestle with a scope of feelings, including dread, uneasiness, dissatisfaction, and bitterness, originating from the vulnerability of their wellbeing, the effect on their day to day routines, and the potential disgrace related with their condition.

   Youths, specifically, may confront extra difficulties connected with self-perception, confidence, and the longing for autonomy. Ongoing sickness can disturb ordinary formative achievements, prompting close to home battles as youngsters attempt to explore their personality and social connections. The close to home effect stretches out to guardians and parental figures, who might encounter sensations of culpability, stress, and stress over their youngster's prosperity and future.

   Mental help, including guiding and psychological well-being administrations, assumes a crucial part in tending to these personal difficulties. Establishing a steady climate that energizes open correspondence and gives assets to adapting is vital for the close to home prosperity of pediatric patients and their families.

3. **Social Seclusion and Shame:**
Constant disease in pediatric patients can add to social seclusion and the potential for defamation, as youngsters might confront difficulties in taking part in average social exercises or might be seen diversely by their friends. School participation might be disturbed because of clinical arrangements or hospitalizations, prompting a feeling of rejection from typical social collaborations. Actual impediments forced by the persistent sickness might additionally add to sensations of seclusion.

Shame can emerge from errors or confusions about the kid's condition, prompting social difficulties in school, local area settings, or even inside more distant family circles. Tending to social confinement and fighting disgrace require a coordinated exertion from guardians, instructors, and medical services suppliers to advance grasping, inclusivity, and consciousness of the interesting necessities of youngsters with persistent sicknesses.

4. **Influence on Relational peculiarities:**
The presence of persistent sickness in a pediatric patient significantly affects relational peculiarities, impacting connections, jobs, and obligations inside the family. Guardians frequently accept the job of essential parental figures, overseeing clinical arrangements, organizing medicines, and offering profound help. Kin might encounter shifts in consideration and assets, possibly prompting sensations of disdain, responsibility, or nervousness.

The monetary strain related with dealing with an ongoing disease, including clinical costs, exceptional gear, and possible loss of pay due to providing care liabilities, can additionally add to family stress. Adjusting the necessities of the youngster with the ongoing disease close by those of other relatives turns into a sensitive shuffling act.

Family-focused care, which includes medical services suppliers perceiving and tending to the effect of constant disease on the whole nuclear family, is fundamental. Support administrations, reprieve care, and advising can assist families with exploring these difficulties, encouraging strength and keeping up with solid relational intricacies.

5. **Instructive Difficulties:**
Constant disease frequently presents instructive difficulties for pediatric patients, influencing their scholarly presentation, participation, and generally instructive experience. Continuous hospitalizations or clinical arrangements might prompt missed school days, influencing a youngster's capacity to stay aware of the educational program.

Actual impediments or mental debilitations related with the constant

disease might require instructive facilities and individualized help.
Teachers and school executives assume a critical part in tending to these difficulties by working cooperatively with medical services suppliers and guardians to make custom fitted training plans. Individualized Training Projects (IEPs) or 504 plans can assist with guaranteeing that the kid gets the fundamental help, facilities, and assets to amplify their instructive potential while dealing with the requests of their ongoing disease.

6. **Monetary Strain:**

The monetary strain related with constant sickness can put a critical weight on pediatric patients and their families. Clinical costs, including prescriptions, medicines, hospitalizations, and specific gear, can amass quickly. Extra expenses might emerge from home adjustments, transportation to clinical arrangements, and likely loss of pay due to providing care liabilities.

Admittance to complete medical care, monetary help projects, and local area assets becomes essential in mitigating the monetary weight. Families confronting monetary strain may likewise profit from advising administrations that give direction on planning, monetary preparation, and getting to accessible encouraging groups of people.

7. **Parental figure Burnout:**

The obligations related with really focusing on a kid with a constant sickness can prompt guardian burnout — a condition of physical, profound, and mental depletion. Guardians frequently shuffle numerous jobs, from overseeing clinical arrangements to organizing treatments and offering profound help. The consistent cautiousness and the unusual idea of constant disease can add to persistent pressure.

Perceiving guardian burnout and executing procedures to address it are fundamental for keeping up with the prosperity of both the parental figure and the pediatric patient. Rest care, support gatherings, and admittance to emotional well-being administrations for parental figures are basic parts of a far reaching care plan that focuses on the soundness of the whole family.

8. **Influence on Future Preparation:**

The presence of a constant sickness in a pediatric patient can impact future anticipating both the individual and the family. Long haul contemplations might incorporate choices about schooling, profession ways, and autonomous living. The vulnerability encompassing the direction of the constant disease might prompt extra pressure while thinking about the kid's future.

Medical services suppliers, as a team with families, assume an essential part in working with conversations about future preparation. This might include investigating professional open doors, addressing expected changes to grown-up care, and laying out a steady organization that can help with exploring the difficulties related with the youngster's developing medical services needs.

9. **Flexibility and Survival techniques:**
   While the effect of constant sickness on pediatric patients and families is certainly difficult, numerous people and families exhibit exceptional versatility and utilize successful survival techniques. Flexibility includes the capacity to adjust decidedly to misfortune, and families frequently foster qualities and survival strategies that empower them to explore the intricacies of persistent ailment.

   Survival techniques might incorporate looking for social help, participating in remedial exercises, getting to psychological wellness administrations, and effectively partaking in backing and encouraging groups of people. Empowering the improvement of versatility and giving assets to adapting is a vital part of pediatric medical care that recognizes the qualities of people and families confronting ongoing ailment.

10. **The Job of Pediatric Medical services Suppliers:**

Pediatric medical services suppliers assume a focal part in tending to the diverse effect of constant sickness on pediatric patients and families. Past clinical administration, successful correspondence, daily reassurance, and cooperation with multidisciplinary groups are vital parts of far reaching care. Medical services suppliers should recognize the psychosocial parts of persistent ailment, effectively pay attention to the worries of patients and families, and give assets to adapting and support.

Joining of psychosocial administrations, including social work, youngster life subject matter experts, and psychological well-being experts, into pediatric medical care groups is fundamental. These experts contribute aptitude in tending to close to home and social difficulties, encouraging versatility, and working with admittance to local area assets. By taking on a comprehensive methodology that envelops both the clinical and psychosocial aspects of persistent disease, pediatric medical services suppliers add to the prosperity of the whole nuclear family.

8.2 Addressing Emotional and Social Challenges

Tending to close to home and social difficulties is a basic part of far reaching medical care, especially with regards to people confronting persistent disease. The profound and social components of wellbeing are interconnected, affecting prosperity and personal satisfaction.

This investigation dives into the significance of tending to profound and social difficulties in medical services, analyzing the effect on people, families, and networks, and featuring methodologies and mediations that add to comprehensive consideration.

1. **The Interconnectedness of Close to home and Social Prosperity:**
Close to home and social prosperity are complicatedly associated, affecting and forming each other in powerful ways. Profound wellbeing includes a singular's capacity to comprehend and deal with their feelings, adapt to pressure, and keep an uplifting perspective on life. Social prosperity, then again, includes the nature of connections, social encouraging groups of people, and the feeling of having a place inside networks.
The exchange among close to home and social prosperity is especially clear even with difficulties like ongoing sickness. People wrestling with medical issue might encounter a scope of feelings, including uneasiness, melancholy, and dread, which can influence their capacity to socially lock in. On the other hand, a vigorous social emotionally supportive network can act as a cushion against close to home trouble, encouraging flexibility and adding to positive psychological wellness results.

2. **Effect of Persistent Sickness on Profound and Social Prosperity:**
Ongoing sickness can essentially influence close to home and social prosperity, presenting a bunch of difficulties that people and families should explore. The close to home cost of dealing with an ongoing condition might incorporate sensations of disappointment, pain, vulnerability about the future, and the pressure of adapting to side effects and medicines. Socially, people with persistent diseases might encounter separation, shame, and interruptions to connections as they adjust to the requests of their medical issue.
For families, the close to home effect reaches out to parental figures who might encounter guardian burnout, stress, and profound weariness. The elements inside the nuclear family can be impacted, and the public activities of both the impacted individual and their relatives might be changed as they battle with the intricacies of persistent disease.

3. **Significance of Basic encouragement:**
Perceiving the significance of basic encouragement is crucial in tending to the difficulties related with persistent ailment. Everyday reassurance includes furnishing people with a place of refuge to communicate their sentiments, approving their encounters, and offering sympathy and understanding. For people confronting ongoing ailment, approaching basic reassurance can fundamentally influence their capacity to adapt to the profound weight of their condition.
Medical care suppliers assume a critical part in offering daily encouragement by cultivating open correspondence, effectively paying attention to patients' interests, and giving assets to psychological wellness

administrations when required. Furthermore, support gatherings, peer mentorship projects, and guiding administrations add to establishing a strong climate that recognizes and addresses the inner difficulties related with ongoing disease.

4. **Social Encouraging groups of people:**
Social encouraging groups of people act as an imperative asset in moderating the effect of persistent disease on both profound and social prosperity. These organizations can incorporate relatives, companions, local gatherings, and medical services experts. Solid social help is related with better wellbeing results, expanded flexibility, and worked on personal satisfaction for people confronting constant circumstances.

Relatives and companions give a primary layer of social help by offering down to earth help, friendship, and close to home consolation. Peer support gatherings, where people confronting comparable wellbeing difficulties can interface and offer encounters, assume a significant part in building a feeling of local area and diminishing sensations of disconnection. Medical services experts add to social help by encouraging cooperative connections, working with admittance to local area assets, and advancing a patient-focused approach that recognizes the significance of the singular's social setting.

5. **Techniques for Tending to Personal Difficulties:**
Tending to inner difficulties related with persistent sickness requires a complex methodology that envelops different procedures and mediations. One key component shows restraint training, giving people data about their condition, treatment choices, and techniques for self-administration. At the point when people have a far reaching comprehension of their wellbeing, they might feel more engaged and in charge, decreasing nervousness and vulnerability.

Integrating psychological well-being screenings into routine medical services appraisals permits medical services suppliers to distinguish personal difficulties right off the bat. Standard registrations with psychological wellness experts, like clinicians or instructors, give people a committed space to examine their close to home prosperity, foster survival techniques, and get remedial help.

Care and unwinding methods, like contemplation and profound breathing activities, are viable apparatuses for overseeing pressure and advancing close to home prosperity. Coordinating these practices into medical care plans can add to an all encompassing methodology that tends to both the physical and close to home parts of ongoing disease.

6. **Advancing Social Consideration and Lessening Shame:**
Advancing social consideration and lessening shame are fundamental parts of tending to the social difficulties related with ongoing sickness.

Disgrace can emerge from confusions or errors about unambiguous ailments, prompting separation and social prohibition. Endeavors to bring issues to light, instruct networks, and encourage a culture of sympathy add to decreasing disgrace and establishing more comprehensive conditions.

Local area commitment programs, support gatherings, and backing drives assume an essential part in advancing social consideration. By making spaces where people with persistent sicknesses can associate, share encounters, and backer for their necessities, these drives add to building steady networks that perceive and esteem the commitments, everything being equal, no matter what their wellbeing status.

7. **Instructive and Working environment Facilities:**
   Instructive and working environment facilities are fundamental in working with social support for people with constant diseases. In instructive settings, joint effort between medical care suppliers, teachers, and families can prompt the improvement of Individualized Schooling Projects (IEPs) or 504 plans that address the remarkable necessities of understudies with constant circumstances. These facilities might remember adaptability for participation, extra help administrations, and adjustments to the educational plan to guarantee instructive achievement.

   Likewise, in the work environment, sensible facilities, for example, adaptable plans for getting work done, alterations to the actual climate, or acclimations to work liabilities can empower people with persistent ailments to partake completely and flourish in their expert lives. Establishing conditions that focus on inclusivity and oblige different wellbeing needs is vital to tending to social difficulties related with persistent sickness.

8. **Enabling People through Self-Support:**
   Enabling people to become advocates for their own prosperity is a groundbreaking system in tending to both profound and social difficulties. Self-backing includes people effectively communicating their requirements, inclinations, and concerns, encouraging a feeling of organization and command over their medical care venture. Medical services suppliers can assume a part in building self-support abilities by giving data, empowering questions, and including people in shared dynamic about their consideration.

   Supporting people in creating powerful relational abilities is a critical part of self-backing. This incorporates articulating their wellbeing needs, communicating concerns, and working together with medical services groups to make care designs that line up with their objectives and values.

   Enabled self-support adds to expanded certainty, further developed correspondence with medical services suppliers, and a more prominent feeling of command over the close to home and social components of residing with an ongoing disease.

9. **Socially Equipped Consideration:**
Socially skilled consideration recognizes the assorted social foundations, convictions, and practices of people and perceives the effect of culture on close to home and social prosperity. Medical care suppliers who are socially equipped take part in aware and comprehensive works on, taking into account the social setting of people with persistent diseases. This approach is fundamental in addressing likely social boundaries to looking for basic encouragement and partaking in friendly exercises.

Socially able consideration includes grasping the social subtleties of well-being convictions, relational intricacies, and correspondence styles. It additionally stresses the significance of including socially important encouraging groups of people, like local area pioneers, strict pioneers, or socially unambiguous associations, in the consideration cycle. By furnishing care that regards and lines up with people's social foundations, medical services suppliers add to a more comprehensive and comprehensive way to deal with tending to profound and social difficulties.

10. **Cooperative Consideration Models:**

Cooperative consideration models that coordinate medical care suppliers, psychological well-being experts, social specialists, and local area assets add to a far reaching approach in tending to profound and social difficulties. These models perceive the interconnectedness of profound and social prosperity and accentuate the significance of cooperative endeavors across medical services disciplines.

In cooperative consideration models, medical services suppliers cooperate to foster coordinated care designs that address both the physical and close to home parts of constant sickness. Emotional wellness experts team up with clinical groups to give convenient mediations and backing. Social laborers assume an imperative part in associating people with local area assets, exploring social difficulties, and pushing for the all encompassing necessities of patients.

8.3 Success Stories in Coping and Support

Examples of overcoming adversity in adapting and support inside the domain of medical services give motivation and important bits of knowledge into the versatility of people confronting difficulties like constant sickness. These accounts feature the groundbreaking force of successful ways of dealing with especially difficult times, powerful emotionally supportive networks, and the cooperative endeavors of medical services suppliers, families, and networks.

Looking at examples of overcoming adversity in adapting and support offers a focal point through which we can comprehend the elements that add to positive results and the manners by which people explore their medical care ventures.

1. **Individual Strengthening through Instruction:**
   One example of overcoming adversity rotates around the extraordinary effect of schooling and individual strengthening. People who effectively look for data about their medical issue, therapy choices, and self-administration systems frequently experience an increased feeling of command over their prosperity. By becoming educated advocates for their own wellbeing, these people are better prepared to simply decide, participate in shared decision-production with medical services suppliers, and effectively partake in their consideration.

   For instance, an individual determined to have a constant condition might leave on an excursion of self-schooling, going to help gatherings, getting to respectable web-based assets, and interfacing with backing associations. This obligation to learning enables people to explore the intricacies of their wellbeing, pose informed inquiries during clinical arrangements, and settle on way of life decisions that line up with their treatment plans. Individual strengthening through training turns into a foundation of effective adapting and cultivates a positive mentality notwithstanding misfortune.

2. **Peer Encouraging groups of people and Shared Encounters:**
   The force of companion encouraging groups of people is clear in examples of overcoming adversity where people confronting comparable wellbeing challenges meet up to share encounters, bits of knowledge, and support. Interfacing with other people who comprehend the subtleties of living with a particular condition makes a feeling of local area and decreases sensations of detachment. Peer encouraging groups of people frequently prosper through help gatherings, online discussions, or local area associations devoted to a specific medical problem.

   In these examples of overcoming adversity, people find comfort in realizing they are in good company in their excursion. They trade viable methods for overseeing side effects, talk about ways of dealing with hardship or stress, and proposition consistent reassurance. The common encounters inside these organizations establish a strong climate where people feel comprehended, approved, and inspired to continue on. Peer encouraging groups of people represent the strength got from aggregate flexibility and the extraordinary effect of shared encounters in exploring the difficulties of persistent ailment.

3. **Comprehensive Ways to deal with Psychological wellness:**
   Examples of overcoming adversity in adapting frequently underscore the significance of tending to psychological wellness as a vital part of

generally prosperity. People who consolidate comprehensive ways to deal with psychological well-being, like care, reflection, and advising, share accounts of worked on close to home flexibility and survival strategies.

These practices add to a positive outlook, decreased feelings of anxiety, and a more adjusted way to deal with dealing with the close to home parts of constant disease.

For example, an individual dealing with an ongoing condition could integrate care procedures into their everyday daily practice, encouraging a more prominent feeling of mindfulness and acknowledgment. Care rehearses, combined with guiding or treatment, give instruments to explore the close to home high points and low points related with persistent ailment. Examples of overcoming adversity highlight the extraordinary effect of focusing on psychological wellness, representing that comprehensive prosperity is a vital consider accomplishing positive results.

4. **Guardian Versatility and Backing:**

Examples of overcoming adversity in adapting stretch out past people confronting persistent sickness to incorporate the parental figures who assume a significant part in offering help. Parental figures frequently explore complex obligations, from organizing clinical arrangements to offering everyday encouragement and overseeing day to day undertakings. Examples of overcoming adversity feature the flexibility of guardians who find strength through encouraging groups of people, taking care of oneself practices, and powerful correspondence with medical services groups.

A guardian's process could include joining parental figure support gatherings, getting to rest care, and learning powerful correspondence techniques to team up with medical services suppliers. These accounts underscore the extraordinary force of parental figure versatility and the significance of perceiving and tending to the one of a kind difficulties looked by the people who offer help to people with persistent diseases. Through strong organizations and taking care of oneself practices, guardians contribute fundamentally to positive results and worked on personal satisfaction for both themselves and the people they care for.

5. **Local area Commitment and Backing:**

Examples of overcoming adversity frequently rise out of people who draw in with their networks, advocate for mindfulness, and add to drives pointed toward working on the existences of those with persistent sicknesses. Backing endeavors might include sharing individual encounters, taking part in mindfulness crusades, or advocating strategy changes to improve medical care availability and emotionally supportive networks.

A singular's process could incorporate turning into a representative for a specific medical issue, sorting out local area occasions, or utilizing virtual entertainment to bring issues to light. These examples of overcoming adversity highlight the extraordinary effect of local area commitment and promotion, showing the way that people can impact positive change in their own lives as well as in the more extensive setting of medical care.

6. **Flexibility in Adjusting to Change:**

Examples of overcoming adversity in adapting frequently feature the flexibility of people in adjusting to the progressions achieved by constant ailment. This flexibility includes tracking down better approaches to seek after objectives, conform to modified everyday schedules, and embrace a reclassified feeling of business as usual. Versatile people share accounts of finding stowed away qualities, creating adaptability, and developing an outlook that embraces change as a piece of their excursion.

For instance, somebody determined to have a persistent condition could turn their profession, investigate new side interests, or foster savvy fixes to defeat actual impediments. These examples of overcoming adversity underscore the extraordinary force of strength, showing that versatility and a positive outlook contribute essentially to exploring the difficulties presented by persistent sickness.

7. **Cooperative Consideration and Patient-Focused Approaches:**

Examples of overcoming adversity frequently underscore the significance of cooperative consideration models and patient-focused approaches in accomplishing positive results. People who effectively draw in with medical services suppliers, partake in shared navigation, and add to the advancement of their consideration designs frequently report further developed fulfillment with their medical care encounters.

In these examples of overcoming adversity, people team up with medical services groups to tailor therapy designs that line up with their objectives and values. They effectively impart their inclinations, express worries, and work along with medical care suppliers to address the extraordinary parts of their wellbeing process. Patient-focused approaches feature the extraordinary effect of engaging people to be dynamic members in their consideration, adding to positive results and a feeling of organization in overseeing ongoing disease.

8. **Using Innovation for Help:**

Examples of overcoming adversity in adapting frequently consolidate the use of innovation to improve backing and self-administration. People influence portable applications, wearable gadgets, and online stages to screen wellbeing measurements, access instructive assets, and associate with virtual help networks. The coordination of innovation gives people devices to participate in their medical services, cultivating a feeling of strengthening and network effectively.

For example, somebody dealing with a constant condition could utilize a cell phone application to follow side effects, set drug updates, or partake in virtual care group gatherings. Examples of overcoming adversity feature the extraordinary effect of innovation as an empowering agent of self-administration and backing, outlining how people can use advanced instruments to improve their medical care insight.

9. **Inventive Articulation and Remedial Outlets:**
Examples of overcoming adversity frequently include people who channel their encounters with ongoing disease into imaginative articulation and restorative outlets. Participating in exercises like craftsmanship, music, composing, or different types of imaginative articulation fills in for of handling feelings, encouraging self-revelation, and tracking down source for self-articulation.

For instance, somebody living with a constant condition could share their process through composing a blog, making workmanship that mirrors their encounters, or creating music that addresses their profound excursion. These examples of overcoming adversity feature the groundbreaking force of inventiveness as a helpful instrument, showing the way that people can track down comfort, therapy, and strengthening through different types of imaginative articulation.

10. **Developing a Positive Steady Climate:**

Examples of overcoming adversity highlight the significance of developing a positive and steady climate, both at home and inside more extensive groups of friends. People who encircle themselves with figuring out relatives, companions, and partners frequently report a more uplifting perspective and further developed survival techniques. The formation of a steady biological system contributes fundamentally to the general prosperity of people confronting constant disease.

In these examples of overcoming adversity, people effectively impart their necessities to their encouraging groups of people, cultivating a climate where open discourse and sympathy flourish. Developing a positive emotionally supportive network includes teaching friends and family about the condition, defining limits when required, and elevating a cooperative way to deal with overseeing wellbeing challenges. Examples of overcoming adversity feature the extraordinary effect of a positive and steady climate on people's capacity to adapt and flourish despite persistent sickness.

CHAPTER 9

Advances in Pediatric Nephrology Research

Progresses in pediatric nephrology research have essentially added to how we might interpret kidney-related messes in youngsters, prompting further developed diagnostics, treatment procedures, and in general quiet results. The field of pediatric nephrology envelops a great many circumstances, including inborn irregularities, hereditary problems, procured kidney infections, and renal transplantation. This investigation dives into key areas of progression in pediatric nephrology research, featuring forward leaps that have molded the scene of care for youngsters with kidney-related conditions.

1. **Hereditary Revelations and Accuracy Medication:**
   One of the remarkable advances in pediatric nephrology research lies in the domain of hereditary revelations and the use of accuracy medication. With progressions in genomic advances, analysts have recognized various hereditary transformations related with pediatric kidney problems.
   These disclosures have not just extended how we might interpret the hereditary premise of conditions, for example, innate nephrotic disorder and polycystic kidney sickness yet have additionally prepared for more designated and customized therapy draws near.
   Accuracy medication in pediatric nephrology includes fitting treatment systems in view of a person's hereditary cosmetics, considering more precise determinations and redid remedial mediations. For instance, distinguishing explicit hereditary transformations related with specific types of nephrotic disorder might impact the selection of meds, possibly further developing treatment adequacy and limiting unfriendly impacts. This change in outlook towards accuracy medication addresses a huge step in giving more individualized and viable consideration for youngsters with kidney problems.

2. **Progresses in Imaging Advances:**

   In the domain of diagnostics, there have been important advances in imaging innovations for surveying pediatric kidney problems. Painless imaging modalities, for example, attractive reverberation imaging (X-ray) and high level ultrasound methods, offer point by point perception of the kidneys and encompassing designs. These advances give clinicians important data for diagnosing inherent abnormalities, surveying kidney capability, and checking illness movement.

   For example, contrast-improved ultrasound and practical X-ray methods consider a more extensive assessment of renal blood stream and tissue perfusion. This can be especially pivotal in surveying kidney capability and identifying anomalies in pediatric patients. These advances in imaging advances upgrade analytic precision as well as add to limiting the requirement for obtrusive strategies in pediatric nephrology, working on the general insight for youthful patients.

3. **Novel Restorative Methodologies:**

   Research in pediatric nephrology has prompted the improvement of novel remedial methodologies for overseeing different kidney problems in youngsters. One prominent model is the rise of designated biologic treatments for explicit types of glomerulonephritis. Biologics, for example, rituximab, have shown guarantee in regulating the safe reaction and easing back illness movement in pediatric patients with specific immune system kidney problems.

   Furthermore, progressions in pharmacogenomics, the investigation of how hereditary varieties impact drug reaction, have prompted more customized and powerful prescription regimens. Understanding what a youngster's hereditary profile might mean for their reaction to specific prescriptions permits medical care suppliers to tailor therapy plans, improving helpful results while limiting the gamble of unfriendly responses. Besides, progressing research is investigating the capability of regenerative medication and undifferentiated organism treatments for kidney recovery and fix. While still in the beginning phases, these imaginative methodologies hold guarantee for tending to the basic reasons for kidney harm and advancing tissue recovery in pediatric patients with kidney issues.

4. **Biomarkers for Early Location and Observing:**

   The recognizable proof of dependable biomarkers for early recognition and checking of pediatric kidney problems has been a critical focal point of exploration. Biomarkers are quantifiable pointers that mirror the presence or movement of an illness. With regards to pediatric nephrology, scientists have gained ground in distinguishing biomarkers related with conditions like intense kidney injury, constant kidney sickness, and explicit hereditary issues.

For instance, urinary biomarkers, for example, neutrophil gelatinase-related lipocalin (NGAL) and kidney injury atom 1 (KIM-1) have shown guarantee in early identification of intense kidney injury in youngsters. Early recognizable proof of kidney injury considers ideal mediation and the board, possibly forestalling further harm.

In the domain of hereditary kidney issues, the revelation of explicit biomarkers related with specific hereditary changes empowers clinicians to successfully screen illness movement and reaction to treatment more. The joining of biomarkers into clinical practice upgrades the accuracy and idealness of symptomatic and checking processes, eventually further developing results for pediatric patients.

5. **Pediatric Renal Transplantation Advancements:**
Propels in pediatric nephrology research have likewise affected the field of renal transplantation in kids. Worked on comprehension of immunology, contributor beneficiary coordinating, and post-relocate care has added to improved results in pediatric renal transplantation.

One outstanding advancement is the refinement of immunosuppressive regimens to limit the gamble of dismissal while lessening the general weight of immunosuppression on pediatric transfer beneficiaries. This has been especially critical in further developing long haul unite endurance and limiting complexities related with immunosuppressive drugs.

Besides, the investigation of elective hotspots for kidney transplantation, like living-related contributors and imaginative departed giver methodologies, has extended the pool of accessible organs for pediatric beneficiaries. Research in this space plans to address the special difficulties of pediatric transplantation, including the shortage of appropriate givers and the requirement for size-matched organs for developing beneficiaries.

6. **Propels in Pediatric Dialysis The board:**
Pediatric nephrology research has added to progresses in the administration of dialysis in youngsters with end-stage renal sickness (ESRD). Nonstop renal substitution treatment (CRRT), a type of dialysis that gives persistent blood sanitization, has acquired conspicuousness in pediatric settings. This methodology offers more noteworthy hemodynamic security and liquid control, making it appropriate for fundamentally sick youngsters with intense kidney injury.

Additionally, research has zeroed in on improving the conveyance of peritoneal dialysis (PD) in pediatric patients. Developments in PD arrangements, catheter innovation, and liquid administration methodologies mean to upgrade the productivity and bearableness of PD in kids, offering a practical option in contrast to hemodialysis.

Also, progressions in locally established peritoneal dialysis programs engage families to effectively partake in their youngster's consideration, advancing more prominent adaptability and working on the general personal satisfaction for pediatric patients requiring dialysis.

7. **Telemedicine and Remote Checking:**
The combination of telemedicine and remote observing advancements has arisen as a huge headway in pediatric nephrology, particularly with regards to continuous patient consideration and follow-up. Telemedicine works with virtual interviews, permitting medical services suppliers to remotely evaluate patients, examine therapy plans, and screen illness movement.

For pediatric patients with persistent kidney conditions, telemedicine offers a helpful and open method for keeping up with customary subsequent arrangements, lessening the requirement for regular emergency clinic visits. Remote checking advances, including wearable gadgets and versatile wellbeing applications, empower ongoing following of significant wellbeing measurements, enabling both medical care suppliers and families in overseeing pediatric kidney problems.

8. **Multi-disciplinary Consideration Models:**

Pediatric nephrology research has highlighted the significance of multi-disciplinary consideration models that include cooperation between nephrologists, pediatricians, specialists, nutritionists, clinicians, and different trained professionals. Perceiving the complicated idea of pediatric kidney problems, multi-disciplinary consideration models mean to give far reaching and all encompassing consideration to address the different requirements of pediatric patients.

These cooperative methodologies include normal group gatherings, shared care plans, and open correspondence among experts to guarantee that every part of a youngster's wellbeing is thought of. For instance, a youngster with constant kidney infection might profit from the mastery of a nutritionist to address dietary requirements, a clinician to help close to home prosperity, and a nephrologist to oversee clinical parts of the condition. Multi-disciplinary consideration models upgrade the general nature of care and add to further developed results for pediatric patients.

9.1 Current Trends in Pediatric Nephrology Research

Latest things in pediatric nephrology research mirror the dynamic and advancing nature of the field, with progressing endeavors to extend how we might interpret kidney-related conditions in youngsters and work on symptomatic and restorative methodologies.

This investigation digs into key patterns in pediatric nephrology research, revealing insight into late advancements that hold guarantee for propelling attention and results for pediatric patients with kidney issues.

1. **Accuracy Medication and Genomic Exploration:**
   One of the noticeable patterns in pediatric nephrology research rotates around accuracy medication and genomic research. The ID of hereditary elements related with different pediatric kidney issues has seen critical improvement. Scientists are utilizing progressed genomic advancements to disentangle the hereditary premise of conditions like inherent abnormalities of the kidney and urinary parcel (CAKUT), nephrotic condition, and acquired renal problems.

   This pattern goes past simply recognizing hereditary transformations; it includes understanding how explicit hereditary variations impact illness vulnerability, movement, and reaction to treatment. The objective is to move towards additional designated and customized mediations in light of a person's hereditary profile. This approach holds extraordinary potential for fitting treatment plans, anticipating illness directions, and streamlining restorative results in pediatric nephrology.

2. **Biomarkers for Early Discovery and Anticipation:**
   The mission for dependable biomarkers for early identification and guess keeps on being a point of convergence in pediatric nephrology research. Distinguishing biomarkers related with explicit kidney conditions considers prior and more precise finding, empowering ideal intercession and further developed results.

   Scientists are investigating various biomarkers in pee and blood tests that can act as marks of kidney wellbeing or the presence of explicit circumstances. For example, novel biomarkers for intense kidney injury (AKI) are being explored to work with early discovery and mediation in pediatric patients, possibly forestalling the movement of kidney harm.

   In addition, the utilization of biomarkers with regards to hereditary kidney problems adds to observing sickness movement and foreseeing complexities, giving significant experiences to clinicians in fitting therapy designs and expecting the exceptional requirements of every patient.

3. **Immunology and Resistant Tweak:**
   Progressions in how we might interpret the safe framework and its job in pediatric kidney problems have prompted expanded center around immunology and resistant balance in research. Immune system kidney sicknesses, like glomerulonephritis and lupus nephritis, are regions where scientists are investigating creative immunomodulatory treatments to address the basic safe dysregulation.

   Biologic treatments focusing on unambiguous parts of the safe framework, like B cells, Lymphocytes, and cytokines, are being explored for their viability in adjusting the resistant reaction and decreasing aggravation in pediatric patients with immune system kidney problems. These treatments mean to accomplish sickness abatement, forestall backslides, and limit the requirement for long haul immunosuppression, consequently working on the general personal satisfaction for impacted kids.

4. **Man-made consciousness and AI Applications:**
The combination of man-made reasoning (man-made intelligence) and AI (ML) applications is arising as a groundbreaking pattern in pediatric nephrology research. These advancements offer the possibility to investigate immense datasets, distinguish examples, and settle on expectations that can illuminate clinical choice making and upgrade patient consideration.

With regards to pediatric nephrology, artificial intelligence and ML applications are being investigated for undertakings, for example, picture examination in radiology and pathology, anticipating illness movement in light of patient information, and streamlining treatment proposals. For instance, computer based intelligence calculations might help with deciphering renal imaging studies, giving more effective and precise findings of innate peculiarities or primary anomalies in pediatric patients.

The use of these advances can possibly upset risk delineation, early intercession, and treatment streamlining, at last further developing results for youngsters with kidney problems.

5. **Telehealth and Remote Checking:**
The Coronavirus pandemic has sped up the reception of telehealth and remote checking in medical services, including pediatric nephrology. This pattern is probably going to continue as scientists and clinicians perceive the advantages of virtual consideration for pediatric patients with kidney problems.

Telehealth works with distant discussions, empowering medical care suppliers to direct virtual visits, screen patients' advancement, and address worries without the requirement for in-person arrangements. This is especially beneficial for pediatric patients and their families, decreasing travel loads and expanding admittance to specific consideration.

Remote checking advancements, including wearable gadgets and locally situated observing instruments, consider nonstop following of important wellbeing measurements. This constant information can support the administration of ongoing kidney conditions, aid early recognition of complexities, and enable families to partake in their youngster's consideration effectively.

6. **Pediatric Renal Transplantation Advancements:**
Pediatric renal transplantation stays a basic area of examination, with

progressing endeavors to further develop unite endurance, limit confusions, and grow the pool of accessible organs. Late patterns in this space remember advancements for immunosuppressive regimens, customized ways to deal with contributor beneficiary coordinating, and methodologies to address the one of a kind difficulties of pediatric transfer beneficiaries.

Progressions in desensitization conventions, which diminish the probability of relocate dismissal, are being investigated to extend the giver pool and upgrade similarity. Moreover, research is centered around refining methodologies for living-contributor kidney transplantation in pediatric patients, guaranteeing ideal results while limiting dangers for the two givers and beneficiaries.

Besides, the investigation of xenotransplantation, the utilization of organs from non-human sources, presents a clever road for tending to the deficiency of contributor organs for pediatric transplantation. While this area is still in the beginning phases of examination, the potential for xenotransplantation to upset pediatric renal transplantation is a promising pattern in ebb and flow research.

7. **Patient-Announced Results and Personal satisfaction Measures:**
Perceiving the significance of patient-focused care, latest things in pediatric nephrology research accentuate the joining of patient-detailed results (Geniuses) and proportions of personal satisfaction. Understanding the effect of kidney problems on the day to day routines of pediatric patients and their families is urgent for fitting mediations and streamlining in general prosperity.

Scientists are investigating the turn of events and approval of Star apparatuses intended for pediatric kidney conditions. These apparatuses expect to catch angles, for example, side effect trouble, treatment-related encounters, and the psychosocial effect of kidney problems. By incorporating Stars into clinical practice, medical care suppliers can acquire a more extensive comprehension of the lived encounters of pediatric patients and utilize this data to direct therapy choices and backing administrations.

8. **Worldwide Wellbeing and Wellbeing Variations:**
Tending to worldwide wellbeing variations in pediatric nephrology is acquiring conspicuousness as a basic examination pattern. Variations in admittance to mind, symptomatic assets, and treatment choices exist on a worldwide scale, influencing the results of pediatric patients with kidney issues, especially in underserved networks.

Analysts are examining ways of improving admittance to screening, diagnostics, and treatment for pediatric kidney conditions in low-asset settings. This incorporates the improvement of practical demonstrative apparatuses, preparing programs for medical care suppliers in asset restricted conditions, and drives to bring issues to light about kidney wellbeing.

Moreover, research is investigating the effect of social determinants of wellbeing on pediatric kidney results. Understanding how factors like financial status, schooling, and admittance to preventive consideration impact the predominance and the board of kidney problems in youngsters is significant for creating designated mediations to diminish wellbeing abberations.

9. **Ecological and Way of life Impacts:**

Ongoing patterns in pediatric nephrology research recognize the job of natural and way of life factors in the turn of events and movement of kidney issues in youngsters. This incorporates the effect of natural poisons, like toxins and weighty metals, on kidney wellbeing, as well as the impact of dietary examples and actual work.

Analysts are examining how openness to natural poisons might add to the advancement of kidney sicknesses in pediatric populaces. Understanding the cooperations between hereditary defenselessness and ecological variables can illuminate preventive methodologies and intercessions to diminish the gamble of kidney issues.

In addition, the investigation of way of life impacts, including diet and exercise, is acquiring consideration in pediatric nephrology research. Way of life changes and preventive measures might assume a huge part in overseeing and moderating the effect of specific kidney conditions, particularly those connected with metabolic and provocative variables.

10. **Multi-disciplinary Coordinated effort and Group Based Care:**

The significance of multi-disciplinary coordinated effort and group based care is progressively perceived as a major pattern in pediatric nephrology research. Given the perplexing idea of kidney issues in youngsters, successful administration requires the ability of different medical services experts, including nephrologists, pediatricians, specialists, attendants, dietitians, clinicians, and social laborers.

Research is centered around assessing the results of multi-disciplinary consideration models in pediatric nephrology. Studies evaluate the effect of cooperative methodologies on tolerant fulfillment, treatment adherence, and generally wellbeing results. The objective is to lay out proof based rehearses that focus on far reaching and composed care for pediatric patients with kidney problems.

9.2 Challenges in Translating Research to Clinical Practice

The interpretation of exploration discoveries into clinical practice, frequently alluded to as "seat to-bedside" interpretation, is an intricate and multi-layered process that presents various difficulties across different fields of medication, including pediatric nephrology. While research tries in pediatric nephrology have taken critical steps in understanding kidney problems in youngsters, the excursion from research revelations to reasonable execution in clinical settings is filled with obstacles that require cautious route. This conversation investigates the difficulties related with making an interpretation of pediatric nephrology examination into successful clinical practices.

1. **Intricacy of Pediatric Kidney Issues:**
   Pediatric kidney issues include a wide range of conditions, going from inborn oddities to hereditary problems and obtained infections. The intrinsic intricacy and heterogeneity of these issues represent a significant test in making an interpretation of examination discoveries to clinical practice. Dissimilar to additional direct circumstances, the complicated idea of pediatric nephrology requires nuanced and custom fitted methodologies that think about the special attributes of every patient.
   For instance, a hereditary transformation related with a particular kidney issue might show contrastingly in individual patients, prompting varieties in sickness movement and reaction to therapy. This intricacy requires customized and patient-focused care, making it trying to foster one-size-fits-all clinical mediations got straightforwardly from research results.
2. **Restricted Generalizability of Study Populaces:**
   Many examination concentrates on in pediatric nephrology include explicit patient populaces, frequently enlisted under controlled conditions to address explicit exploration questions. While these examinations contribute important experiences, the restricted generalizability of discoveries to different patient populaces experienced in certifiable clinical settings represents a critical test.
   Clinical practice includes an expansive range of patients with differing socioeconomics, comorbidities, and hereditary foundations. Research led on a somewhat homogeneous gathering of patients may not completely catch the intricacies saw in the more extensive populace. Making an interpretation of such discoveries to assorted patient partners turns into a test, as the materialness of exploration results to various segment bunches stays questionable.
3. **Delay Among Exploration and Execution:**
   The delay between the age of exploration proof and its execution in clinical practice is an unavoidable test in medical care.
   The method involved with leading thorough exploration, acquiring administrative endorsements, and scattering discoveries through distributions

takes time. In this manner, coordinating these discoveries into routine clinical consideration faces unexpected setbacks.

The quick development of clinical information and mechanical progressions further intensifies this test. When certain examination discoveries are prepared for execution, new disclosures might have arisen, prompting a consistent battle to keep clinical practices lined up with the most recent proof. Overcoming any barrier between research headways and their ideal coordination into clinical work processes stays a tenacious test in pediatric nephrology.

4. **Absence of Normalization and Agreement:**
   The shortfall of normalized conventions and agreement rules in pediatric nephrology research adds to difficulties in making an interpretation of examination into clinical practice. While research studies give important experiences, the absence of consistency in philosophies, analytic rules, and treatment conventions hampers the consistent reconciliation of discoveries into normalized clinical methodologies.

   For example, unique exploration studies might utilize changed definitions for illness results, making it trying to lay out all around acknowledged benchmarks for determination and treatment. This absence of normalization muddles endeavors to execute proof based rehearses reliably across various medical services settings and establishments.

5. **Moral and Administrative Contemplations:**
   Moral and administrative contemplations assume a urgent part in the interpretation of pediatric nephrology examination into clinical practice. Research including pediatric populaces requires adherence to rigid moral rules to guarantee the prosperity of weak subjects. While these rules are fundamental for protecting patients, they can likewise obstruct the quick interpretation of exploration discoveries into viable applications.

   Severe administrative cycles, including institutional survey board endorsements and consistence with moral principles, add layers of intricacy to the interpretation interaction. While these shields are basic for patient security, the careful adherence to moral and administrative necessities can bring about defers in carrying out clever mediations and treatments got from research.

6. **Restricted Industry Contribution and Financing:**
   The interpretation of examination discoveries frequently requires cooperation with industry accomplices for the turn of events and commercialization of new diagnostics, medications, or advancements. Notwithstanding, restricted industry association and subsidizing in pediatric nephrology research present critical difficulties in carrying creative mediations from the lab to the facility.

   The moderately little understanding populace and exceptional difficulties related with pediatric kidney problems might stop drug organizations and industry partners from putting resources into innovative work for this particular field. Thus, the interpretation of examination discoveries into substantial clinical arrangements might confront monetary imperatives and asset constraints.

7. **Interdisciplinary Cooperation and Correspondence Obstructions:**
Pediatric nephrology, in the same way as other clinical claims to fame, requires interdisciplinary coordinated effort for exhaustive patient consideration. In any case, correspondence obstructions and storehouses between various disciplines can block the viable interpretation of examination into clinical practice.

Analysts, clinicians, nurture, and partnered medical care experts frequently work inside particular spaces, and laying out viable correspondence channels among these different partners is fundamental. Overcoming any issues between research discoveries and clinical execution requires consistent cooperation and information trade, however these endeavors can be impeded by institutional designs, correspondence holes, and differing levels of examination education among medical care experts.

8. **Protection from Change and Latency in Clinical Practice:**
Protection from change and latency inside clinical practice address imposing difficulties in making an interpretation of examination discoveries into noteworthy systems. Laid out clinical schedules, imbued propensities, and customary ways to deal with patient consideration might oppose mix with novel intercessions got from research.

Clinicians, particularly those with longstanding experience, may display a hesitance to take on new practices, especially in the event that they see them as disturbing laid out work processes or on the other hand in the event that there is an absence of powerful proof supporting the change. Defeating this obstruction and cultivating a culture of constant improvement and versatility inside clinical settings is vital for effective interpretation of investigation into training.

9. **Restricted Patient and Guardian Commitment:**
Patient and parental figure commitment is a urgent part of fruitful interpretation from exploration to clinical practice, especially in pediatric nephrology where the prosperity of youngsters is foremost. Be that as it may, restricted contribution of patients and their families in the examination cycle and lacking correspondence about research discoveries might upset the effective take-up of creative methodologies in clinical consideration.

Guaranteeing that patients and parental figures are educated, taught, and effectively associated with dynamic cycles can improve the interpretation interaction. Engaging families with information about the most recent examination and treatment choices cultivates a cooperative connection between medical care suppliers and those straightforwardly impacted by pediatric kidney problems.

10. **Asset Limitations and Medical services Inconsistencies:**

Asset requirements and medical care differences present critical difficulties in making an interpretation of examination into clinical practice, particularly with regards to pediatric nephrology. Restricted assets, both monetary and infrastructural, in specific medical care settings might hinder the reception of new advances, analytic devices, or therapy modalities got from research.

Besides, medical services variations can bring about inconsistent admittance to imaginative mediations, making a gap in the nature of care gave to various populaces. Spanning these holes requires purposeful endeavors to address fundamental disparities and guarantee that progressions in pediatric nephrology are open to all kids, paying little heed to financial or geological variables.

9.3 Future Directions and Potential Triumphs

The eventual fate of pediatric nephrology holds energizing possibilities as specialists and medical services experts keep on propelling comprehension they might interpret kidney problems in youngsters. Arising innovations, imaginative treatments, and a developing accentuation on customized medication are molding the scene of pediatric nephrology, making ready for expected wins in quiet consideration, results, and by and large personal satisfaction. This conversation investigates future headings and the potential victories that might unfurl in the field of pediatric nephrology.

1. **Accuracy Medication and Customized Treatments:**
   The advancement of accuracy medication is ready to alter the treatment scene for pediatric kidney problems. As how we might interpret the hereditary premise of these circumstances extends, scientists are investigating the potential for custom-made and customized treatments. Accuracy medication includes tweaking treatment plans in light of a person's hereditary cosmetics, considering more designated and viable mediations.

   Later on, hereditary profiling might direct treatment choices, empowering clinicians to choose treatments that are explicitly matched to a kid's hereditary profile. This customized approach can possibly upgrade treatment viability while limiting secondary effects, offering a huge victory in improving patient results in pediatric nephrology.

2. **Progresses in Regenerative Medication:**
   The field of regenerative medication holds guarantee for changing the

treatment of kidney issues in youngsters. Specialists are investigating regenerative treatments, including undifferentiated cell based approaches, to fix and recover harmed kidney tissue. While still in the beginning phases of improvement, these imaginative procedures mean to address the hidden reasons for kidney harm and advance utilitarian recuperation. Regenerative medication might offer new roads for treating innate peculiarities, hereditary problems, and procured kidney sicknesses in pediatric patients. Outcome in this space might actually diminish the requirement for transplantation and long haul dialysis, denoting a victory in giving more feasible and less obtrusive treatment choices for youngsters with kidney problems.

3. **Combination of Computerized reasoning and AI:**

The combination of computerized reasoning (simulated intelligence) and AI (ML) applications is probably going to assume a urgent part in store for pediatric nephrology. These innovations can possibly dissect tremendous measures of clinical information, recognize designs, and give prescient investigation. With regards to pediatric kidney issues, computer based intelligence and ML applications can aid early determination, risk separation, and treatment enhancement.

For instance, computer based intelligence calculations might assist with anticipating sickness movement, taking into consideration ideal intercessions to forestall difficulties. Also, these advances can add to the translation of perplexing imaging studies, helping with the determination of inborn irregularities and other primary anomalies in pediatric kidneys. The effective combination of man-made intelligence and ML can possibly upgrade clinical independent direction, prompting further developed results for youngsters with kidney issues.

4. **Advancement of Novel Biomarkers:**

Progressions in the recognizable proof of biomarkers hold huge commitment for the fate of pediatric nephrology. Analysts are investigating novel biomarkers that can act as early signs of kidney harm, illness movement, and treatment reaction. These biomarkers might be identified in pee or blood tests, giving painless and delicate proportions of kidney wellbeing. The accessibility of solid biomarkers can work with early finding and intercession, possibly forestalling the movement of kidney issues. Checking these biomarkers may likewise help with fitting treatment designs and evaluating the adequacy of restorative mediations. The turn of events and approval of powerful biomarkers address a possible victory in working on the accuracy and practicality of diagnostics and mediations in pediatric nephrology.

5. **Upgraded Telehealth and Remote Observing:**

The encounters acquired during the Coronavirus pandemic have sped up the reception of telehealth and remote observing in medical services, and these patterns are probably going to keep molding the eventual fate of pediatric nephrology. Telehealth works with virtual counsels, empowering medical care suppliers to arrive at pediatric patients and their families, especially those in remote or underserved regions.

Remote checking advancements, including wearable gadgets and versatile wellbeing applications, can enable families to effectively take part in the administration of pediatric kidney problems.

Ongoing following of important wellbeing measurements considers persistent observing and ideal mediations. The expanded openness and comfort gave by telehealth and remote checking can prompt better persistent commitment and results, addressing a victory in extending medical services access and upgrading patient-focused care.

6. **Creative Ways to deal with Pediatric Renal Transplantation:**
The eventual fate of pediatric nephrology remembers progressing headways for renal transplantation, with an emphasis on refining strategies, further developing results, and tending to the special difficulties looked by pediatric transfer beneficiaries. Developments in immunosuppressive regimens plan to work out some kind of harmony between forestalling dismissal and limiting long haul confusions.

Additionally, the investigation of elective hotspots for kidney transplantation, like living-related benefactors and xenotransplantation (utilizing organs from non-human sources), may extend the pool of accessible organs for pediatric beneficiaries. Progress in these undertakings could reduce the shortage of reasonable givers and further develop the drawn out unite endurance rates for pediatric renal transfer beneficiaries, denoting a victory in the field.

7. **Patient-Focused Exploration and Shared Independent direction:**
The fate of pediatric nephrology is progressively centered around tolerant focused research and shared direction. Perceiving the significance of including patients and their families in treatment choices, scientists are underlining the fuse of patient-announced results (Masters) and inclinations in clinical examinations.

Drawing in pediatric patients and their families in shared direction guarantees that treatment plans line up with their qualities, inclinations, and way of life. This approach upgrades the general insight of care and adds to further developed adherence to treatment regimens. The combination of patient-focused research and shared direction addresses a victory in cultivating cooperative and individualized care in pediatric nephrology.

8. **Tending to Medical care Inconsistencies and Worldwide Wellbeing Imbalances:**
The eventual fate of pediatric nephrology includes a coordinated work to

address medical services variations and worldwide wellbeing disparities. Scientists and medical services experts are pursuing creating systems to further develop admittance to mind, analytic assets, and therapy choices for pediatric kidney issues in underserved networks.

This incorporates drives to improve schooling, mindfulness, and preventive consideration in areas with restricted assets. Win in this space would include restricting the hole in medical services results between various populaces, guaranteeing that all youngsters, no matter what their financial status or geological area, approach excellent pediatric nephrology care.

9. **Incorporation of Multidisciplinary Care Models:**

The fate of pediatric nephrology will probably observe an expanded accentuation on multidisciplinary care models. Perceiving the perplexing idea of kidney problems in youngsters, medical services suppliers are embracing cooperative methodologies that include nephrologists, pediatricians, specialists, nutritionists, clinicians, and different trained professionals.

Incorporating skill from different disciplines guarantees thorough and comprehensive consideration, tending to not just the clinical parts of pediatric kidney issues yet in addition the psychosocial and dietary requirements of patients. Progress in executing powerful multidisciplinary care models would address a victory in giving balanced and individualized care for pediatric patients.

10. **Patient Promotion and Local area Commitment:**

As what's in store unfurls, patient backing and local area commitment are supposed to assume an undeniably powerful part in pediatric nephrology. Patient support gatherings, engaged by progressions in correspondence and systems administration, can add to bringing issues to light, advancing exploration, and affecting strategy choices connected with pediatric kidney problems.

Local area commitment drives might include instructive projects, encouraging groups of people, and effort endeavors to guarantee that families and networks are very much informed about kidney wellbeing. The victory in this space lies in building areas of strength for a strong local area that effectively partakes in the headway of pediatric nephrology, pushing for the requirements of youngsters with kidney issues.